Workbook for Bushong's

Radiologic Science for Technologists

Thirteenth Edition

Workbook for Bushong's

Radiologic Science for Technologists

Thirteenth Edition

Prepared by:

Alisha L. Hogan, MS, RT(R)(CT)
Associate Professor
Radiologic Sciences Program Director
Carolinas College of Health Sciences
Charlotte, North Carolina

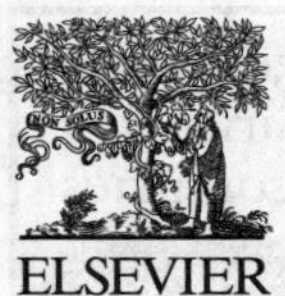

ELSEVIER

Elsevier
3251 Riverport Lane
St. Louis, Missouri 63043

WORKBOOK FOR BUSHONG'S RADIOLOGIC SCIENCE FOR TECHNOLOGISTS, THIRTEENTH EDITION ISBN: 978-0-323-93074-1

For accessibility purposes, images in electronic versions of this book are accompanied by alt-text descriptions provided by Elsevier. For more information, see https://www.elsevier.com/about/accessibility.

Books and Journals published by Elsevier comply with applicable product safety requirements. For any product safety concerns or queries, please contact our authorised representative, Elsevier B.V., at productsafety@elsevier.com or Radarweg 29, 1043 NX Amsterdam, Netherlands.

Publisher's note: Elsevier takes a neutral position with respect to territorial disputes or jurisdictional claims in its published content, including in maps and institutional affiliations.

Notice

Practitioners and researchers must always rely on their own experience and knowledge in evaluating and using any information, methods, compounds or experiments described herein. Because of rapid advances in the medical sciences, in particular, independent verification of diagnoses and drug dosages should be made. To the fullest extent of the law, no responsibility is assumed by Elsevier, authors, editors or contributors for any injury and/or damage to persons or property as a matter of products liability, negligence or otherwise, or from any use or operation of any methods, products, instructions, or ideas contained in the material herein.

Previous editions copyrighted 2021, 2017, 2012 and 2008.

Senior Content Strategist: Meg Benson/Luke Held
Content Development Manager: Danielle Frazier
Senior Content Development Specialist: Sarah Vora
Publishing Services Manager: Deepthi Unni
Project Manager: Haritha Dharmarajan
Cover Designer: Gopalakrishnan Venkatraman

Printed in India at Replika Press Pvt. Ltd.
Plot No. 310-311, EPIP, HSIIDC, Kundli Industrial Park,
Sonipat, Haryana – 131028.

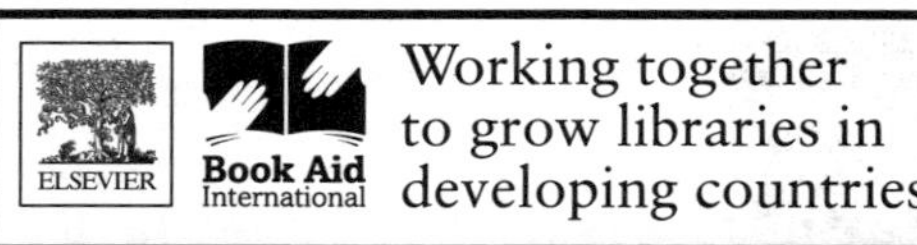

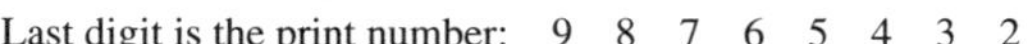
Last digit is the print number: 9 8 7 6 5 4 3 2

Preface

Straightforward and fun, the workbook stimulates discussion while helping students review information and develop the skills necessary to become informed and competent radiologic technologists.

Similar to previous editions, the 13th edition contains worksheets that are organized by topic and numbered according to the textbook chapters. The worksheet numbers and descriptive titles make it easy to find worksheets to test specific topics or coordinate with the major concepts of a textbook chapter; they primarily contain multiple choice questions that can be quickly graded and returned. The answer keys can be found on the Evolve site at http://evolve.elsevier.com.

Each worksheet features "Penguins" to aid in the successful completion of the exercises. The Penguins provide a concise summary of information that is relevant to the exercise questions. Lighthearted and to the point, Penguins make it easier than ever to review major textbook concepts.

As always, Elsevier welcomes your comments about this book or any of our other imaging sciences publications.

The authors especially appreciate your comments regarding any of the material in this volume. Please e-mail me at sbushong@bcm.edu so that together we can make this material even more instructive and "Physics even more Phun."

Contents

PART I: RADIOLOGIC PHYSICS

Chapter 1: Essential Concepts of Radiologic Science
Worksheet 1-1: Nature of Our Surroundings Matter and Energy Sources of Ionizing Radiation, **1**
Worksheet 1-2: Discovery of X-Rays Development of Medical Imaging, **3**
Worksheet 1-3: Reports of Radiation Injury Basic Radiation Protection The Medical Imaging Team, **5**
Worksheet 1-4: Numeric Prefixes, **7**
Worksheet 1-5: Radiologic Units, **9**

Chapter 2: Basic Physics Primer
Worksheet 2-1: Standard Units of Measurement, **11**
Worksheet 2-2: Newton's Laws, **13**
Worksheet 2-3: Mechanics, **15**

Chapter 3: The Structure of Matter
Worksheet 3-1: Centuries of Discovery, **17**
Worksheet 3-2: Fundamental Particles Atomic Structure, **19**
Worksheet 3-3: Atomic Nomenclature Combinations of Atoms, **21**
Worksheet 3-4: Radioactivity, **23**
Worksheet 3-5: Types of Ionizing Radiation, **25**

Chapter 4: Electromagnetic Energy
Worksheet 4-1: Photons, **27**
Worksheet 4-2: Electromagnetic Spectrum, **29**
Worksheet 4-3: Wave-Particle Duality, **31**
Worksheet 4-4: Inverse Square Law, **33**
Worksheet 4-5: X-Ray Photons, **35**
Worksheet 4-6: Matter and Energy, **37**

Chapter 5: Electricity, Magnetism, and Electromagnetism
Worksheet 5-1: Electrostatics, **39**
Worksheet 5-2: Electrodynamics, **41**
Worksheet 5-3: Alternating and Direct Currents, **43**
Worksheet 5-4: Magnetism, **45**
Worksheet 5-5: Electromagnetic Effect Electromagnetic Induction, **47**
Worksheet 5-6: Electromagnetic Devices, **49**
Worksheet 5-7: The Transformer, **51**

PART II: X-RADIATION

Chapter 6: The X-Ray Imaging System
Worksheet 6-1: Operating Console Control of Kilovolt Peak (kVp), **53**
Worksheet 6-2: Operating Console Control of Milliamperage (mA), **55**
Worksheet 6-3: Operating Console Exposure Timers, **57**
Worksheet 6-4: High-Voltage Generator High-Voltage Generation, **59**
Worksheet 6-5: High-Voltage Generator Rectification, **61**

Chapter 7: The X-Ray Tube
Worksheet 7-1: Internal Components The X-Ray Tube Cathode, **63**
Worksheet 7-2: Internal Components The X-Ray Tube Anode, **65**
Worksheet 7-3: X-Ray Tube Failure X-Ray Tube Rating Charts, **67**

Chapter 8: X-Ray Production
Worksheet 8-1: Electron-Target Interactions Characteristic Radiation, **69**
Worksheet 8-2: Electron-Target Interactions Bremsstrahlung Radiation, **71**
Worksheet 8-3: X-Ray Emission Spectrum, **73**
Worksheet 8-4: X-Ray Emission Spectrum Minimum Wavelength, **75**
Worksheet 8-5: X-Ray Emission Spectrum Factors That Affect the X-Ray Emission Spectrum, **77**

Chapter 9: X-Ray Emission
Worksheet 9-1: X-Ray Emission X-Ray Quantity, **79**
Worksheet 9-2: X-Ray Emission X-Ray Quality, **81**
Worksheet 9-3: X-Ray Emission Half-Value Layer, **83**
Worksheet 9-4: X-Ray Emission Filtration, **85**

Chapter 10: X-Ray Interaction With Matter
Worksheet 10-1: X-Ray Interaction With Matter Compton Effect, **87**
Worksheet 10-2: X-Ray Interaction With Matter Photoelectric Effect, **89**
Worksheet 10-3: X-Ray Interaction With Matter Differential Absorption/Atomic Number, **91**
Worksheet 10-4: X-Ray Interaction With Matter Differential Absorption/Mass Density, **93**

PART III: X-RAY IMAGING

Chapter 11: Computed Radiography
Worksheet 11-1: Computed Radiography Image Receptor, **95**
Worksheet 11-2: Computed Radiography Reader, **97**

Chapter 12: Digital Radiography
Worksheet 12-1: Direct Radiography, **99**

Chapter 13: Digital Radiographic Technique
Worksheet 13-1: Spatial Resolution, **101**
Worksheet 13-2: Contrast Resolution Contrast Detail, **103**

Chapter 14: Image Acquisition
Worksheet 14-1: Exposure Time, **105**
Worksheet 14-2: Adjusting for Change in Distance, **107**
Worksheet 14-3: Characteristics of the Imaging System, **109**
Worksheet 14-4: Magnification Radiography, **111**

Chapter 15: Scatter Radiation
Worksheet 15-1: Production of Scatter Radiation, **113**
Worksheet 15-2: Control of Scatter Radiation, **115**
Worksheet 15-3: Radiographic Grids, **117**
Worksheet 15-4: Measuring Grid Performance, **119**
Worksheet 15-5: Types of Grids Use of Grids Grid Selection, **121**

Chapter 16: Digital Image Descriptors and Evaluation
Worksheet 16-1: Image Descriptors, **123**
Worksheet 16-2: Image Quality Tools, **125**

Chapter 17: Radiographic Artifacts
Worksheet 17-1: Digital Radiographic Artifacts, **127**

PART IV: ADVANCED MEDICAL IMAGING

Chapter 18: Mammography
Worksheet 18-1: Mammography, **129**
Worksheet 18-2: Quality Control Team Quality Control Program, **131**

Chapter 19: Fluoroscopy
Worksheet 19-1: Image Intensification, **133**
Worksheet 19-2: Image Monitoring, **135**
Worksheet 19-3: Digital Fluoroscopy, **137**

Chapter 20: Interventional Radiology
Worksheet 20-1: Types of Procedures Basic Principles IR Suite, **141**

Chapter 21: Computed Tomography
Worksheet 21-1: Principles of Operation of CT, **143**
Worksheet 21-2: CT Image Characteristics Image Quality Quality Control, **145**
Worksheet 21-3: Operational CT Modes, **147**

Chapter 22: Tomosynthesis
Worksheet 22-1: Digital Radiographic Tomosynthesis, **151**
Worksheet 22-2: Conventional Tomography, **153**

PART V: MEDICAL IMAGE DISPLAY

Chapter 23: Patient-Image Optimization
Worksheet 23-1: Patient Factors, **155**
Worksheet 23-2: Image Quality Factors, **156**
Worksheet 23-3: Distortion, **158**
Worksheet 23-4: Improving Radiographic Quality, **160**

Chapter 24: Viewing the Medical Image
Worksheet 24-1: Photometric Quantities, **163**

Chapter 25: Medical Image Informatics
Worksheet 25-1: Electronic Programs, **165**

Chapter 26: Digital Display Device
Worksheet 26-1: Digital Display Device Performance Assessment, **167**
Worksheet 26-2: Digital Display Quality Control, **169**

PART VI: THE MEDICAL IMAGE

Chapter 27: Imaging Science
Worksheet 27-1: Computer Applications, **171**
Worksheet 27-2: Computer Applications within Radiology, **173**

Chapter 28: Artificial Intelligence
Worksheet 28-1: Artificial Intelligence, **175**

Chapter 29: Quantum Computing
Worksheet 29-1: Evolution from Classical Physics to Quantum Mechanics, **179**

Chapter 30: Image Perception
Worksheet 30-1: Digital Image Perception, **181**
Worksheet 30-2: Receiver Operating Characteristics Curves, **183**

PART VII: RADIOBIOLOGY

Chapter 31: Human Biology
Worksheet 31-1: Human Radiation Response Composition of the Body, **185**
Worksheet 31-2: Cell Theory, **187**
Worksheet 31-3: Human Cells Tissues and Organs, **189**

Chapter 32: Fundamental Principles of Radiobiology
Worksheet 32-1: Law of Bergonié and Tribondeau Physical Factors That Affect Radiosensitivity, **191**
Worksheet 32-2: Biologic Factors That Affect Radiosensitivity Radiation Dose-Response Relationships, **193**

Chapter 33: Molecular Radiobiology
Worksheet 33-1: Molecular Radiobiology, **195**

Chapter 34: Cellular Radiobiology
Worksheet 34-1: Cellular Radiobiology, **197**

Chapter 35: Deterministic Effects of Radiation
Worksheet 35-1: Acute Radiation Lethality Local Tissue Damage, **199**
Worksheet 35-2: Hematologic Effects Cytogenetic Effects, **201**

Chapter 36: Stochastic Effects of Radiation
Worksheet 36-1: Local Tissue Effects Life Span Shortening Risk Estimates, **203**
Worksheet 36-2: Radiation-Induced Malignancy Total Risk of Malignancy Radiation and Pregnancy, **205**

PART VIII: RADIATION PROTECTION

Chapter 37: Health Physics
Worksheet 37-1: Cardinal Principles of Radiation Protection Dose Limits, **207**

Chapter 38: Designing for Radiation Protection
Worksheet 38-1: Design of X-Ray Apparatus Design of Protective Barriers, **209**
Worksheet 38-2: Radiation Detection and Measurement, **211**

Chapter 39: Radiography/Fluoroscopy Patient Radiation Dose
Worksheet 39-1: Patient Radiation Dose Reduction of Unnecessary Patient Dose, **213**

Chapter 40: Computed Tomography Patient Radiation Dose
Worksheet 40-1: CT Patient Radiation Dose, **215**

Chapter 41: Patient Radiation Dose Management
Worksheet 41-1: Patient Radiation Dose Management, **217**

Chapter 42: Occupational Radiation Dose Management
Worksheet 42-1: Occupational Radiation Dose Management, **219**

Worksheet 1-1
Nature of Our Surroundings
Matter and Energy
Sources of Ionizing Radiation

Some representative radiation levels are as follows:

In Our Daily Lives:

Living next to a nuclear power station	5 μSv/y (0.5 mrem/y)
Cross-country jet flight	20 μSv (2 mrem)
Fallout at the height of atomic weapons testing	50 μSv (5 mrem)
Consumer products (e.g., smoke detectors and watch dials)	30 μSv/y (3 mrem/y)
Natural Background	
Sea level	1 mSv/y (100 mrem/y)
Mountains	5 mSv/y (500 mrem/y)
The Healing Arts	
^{99m}Tc thyroid image	100 μGy_t (10 mrad)
Mean marrow dose	1 mGy_t (100 mrad)
Entrance Skin Exposure	
posterior-anterior chest (PA) examination	100 μGy_a (10 mR)
Panoramic dental x-ray	2 mGy_a (200 mR)
Lumbar spine examination	10 mGy_a/min (1000 mR)
Fluoroscopic examination	40 mGy_a/min (4000 mR/min)
Computed Tomography	
Head examination	40 mGy_t (4000 mrad)
Body examination	20 mGy_t (2000 mrad)
Occupational Dose Limit	
Radiographer	50 mSv/y (5000 mrem/y)
Public	1 mSv/y (100 mrem/y)

MASS IS THE QUANTITY OF MATTER DESCRIBED BY ITS ENERGY EQUIVALENCE.

ENERGY IS THE ABILITY TO DO WORK.

RADIATION IS THE TRANSFER OF ENERGY.

EXERCISES

1. Which of the following items is considered as matter?
   a. Airport surveillance x-rays
   b. Anode heat
   c. Cell phone signals
   d. Light from a movie projector
   e. Wet snow

2. Which of the following is the principal difference between mass and weight?
   a. Mass is measured in pounds (lb); weight is measured in kilograms (kg).
   b. Mass is the equivalence of energy; weight is the force exerted by gravity.
   c. There is no difference; mass and weight are equal.
   d. Weight does not change with position; mass does.
   e. Weight is energy; mass requires gravity.

3. *Energy* is defined as:
   a. A force exerted by a body
   b. Anything that occupies space and has shape
   c. The ability to do work
   d. The degree of gravity
   e. The quantity of matter

4. Which of the following examples *best* represents energy?
   a. A snowman
   b. A thrown snowball
   c. Anode mass
   d. The metal plates in a battery
   e. The terminals of a battery

5. Which of the following is *NOT* an example of potential energy?
   a. Bow and arrow
   b. Mobile x-ray imaging system in motion
   c. Rubber band
   d. Roller coaster
   e. Microwave

6. In Einstein's famous $E = mc^2$ equation, c stands for which of the following?
   a. Acceleration of mass
   b. Force
   c. Mass-energy equivalence
   d. The speed of light
   e. The theory of relativity

7. *Radiation* is:
   a. Energy transferred
   b. Isotropic emission
   c. Kinetic particles
   d. Mass with a charge
   e. Measured in joules

8. The milligray in air (mGya) relates to which of the following?
   a. A dose equivalent
   b. Ions produced in the air
   c. Isotropic emission
   d. Nonionizing radiation
   e. Tissue-absorbed dose

9. Which of the following is an example of electromagnetic radiation?
   a. Alpha radiation
   b. Beta rays
   c. Sound
   d. Ultrasound
   e. Visible light

10. When ionization occurs, which of the following is *true?*
    a. The negative ion is electromagnetic radiation.
    b. The negative ion is the ion pair.
    c. The negative ion is the target atom.
    d. The positive ion is electromagnetic.
    e. The positive ion is the resulting atom.

11. X-rays are *most* like:
    a. Alpha rays
    b. Beta rays
    c. Diagnostic ultrasound
    d. Gamma rays
    e. Radio waves

12. Which of the following is the largest source of human exposure to man-made radiation?
    a. Cosmic rays
    b. Medical diagnostic radiation
    c. Nuclear power–generating stations
    d. Radioactive fallout
    e. Radioactive materials in consumer products

13. What is the approximate annual effective dose from natural environmental radiation at sea level?
    a. 50 μSv/y (5 mrem/y)
    b. 100 μSv/y (10 mrem/y)
    c. 500 μSv/y (50 mrem/y)
    d. 1 mSv/y (100 mrem/y)
    e. 5 mSv/y (500 mrem/y)

14. Which of the following results in the highest annual radiation dose?
    a. Cosmic rays
    b. Diagnostic x-rays
    c. Microwave radiation
    d. Nuclear power
    e. Radiation from inside the Earth

15. Which of the following is the largest source of background radiation to each of us annually?
    a. Consumer products
    b. Exposure to radon
    c. Microwave oven radiation
    d. Radioactive fallout radiation
    e. Radioisotopes in nuclear medicine

16. Which of the following is a unit of mass?
    a. Joule
    b. Kilogram
    c. mrad
    d. Pound
    e. Volt

17. Which of the following is ionizing electromagnetic radiation?
    a. Beta rays
    b. Gamma rays
    c. Microwaves
    d. Radio waves
    e. Ultrasound

18. Which of the following is a unit of energy?
    a. Joule
    b. Kilogram
    c. mrad
    d. Pound
    e. Volt

Worksheet 1-2
Discovery of X-Rays
Development of Medical Imaging

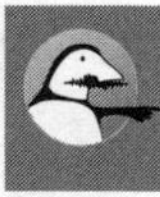

- X-rays were discovered in 1895 by Roentgen.
- The cadmium tungstate ($CdWO_4$) radiographic intensifying screen was developed by Edison and was first used in 1898.
- Clarence Dally, who was an assistant to Edison, died of radiation injuries in 1904.
- In 1913 Coolidge developed the modern heated filament x-ray tube.
- The National Council on Radiation Protection (NCRP) reduced the occupational dose limit to 50 mSv/y in 1957.
- The image-intensifier tube became available in the early 1960s.
- Diagnostic ultrasound was introduced in the early 1960s.
- Computed tomography appeared in 1972.
- Magnetic resonance imaging was introduced for clinical use in 1980.
- The first federal imaging regulation—the Mammography Quality Standards Act—was passed in 1992.
- The first all-digital department of radiology (Baltimore Veterans Affairs Medical Center) opened in 1993.
- Solid-state digital image receptors were introduced in 1996.
- The Radiological Society of North America presented the first annual showing of Integrating the Healthcare Environment in 1997.
- Multislice helical computed tomography appeared in 1998.
- Digital mammography was approved by the US Food and Drug Administration in 2000.
- Positron emission tomography was assumed a role in clinical practice in 2002.
- Sixty four–slice helical computed tomography was offered in 2004 by several vendors.
- Dual-source computed tomography was introduced in 2005 (Siemens).
- Three hundred twenty–slice helical computed tomography is now available (Toshiba).

EXERCISES

1. What was the device with which Roentgen discovered x-rays?
   a. Anode tube
   b. Coolidge tube
   c. Crookes tube
   d. Geissler tube
   e. Snook interrupterless transformer

2. The phosphor that Roentgen used in early experiments with x-rays was which of the following?
   a. Barium platinocyanide
   b. Cadmium tungstate
   c. Calcium tungstate
   d. Rare earth
   e. Zinc cadmium sulfide

3. How are x-ray tube voltages measured?
   a. Kilovolt
   b. Megavolt
   c. Microvolt
   d. Millivolt
   e. Volt

4. Which of the following early pioneers developed the fluoroscope?
   a. Alexander G. Bell
   b. J.J. Thomson
   c. Thomas Edison
   d. Wilhelm Roentgen
   e. William Crookes

5. Who first applied x-ray beam collimation and filtration in medical imaging?
   a. Wilhelm Roentgen
   b. William Coolidge
   c. William Crookes
   d. William Longfellow
   e. William Rollins

6. Which of the following is the type of x-ray tube that is used today?
   a. Coolidge tube
   b. Crookes tube
   c. Geissler tube
   d. Leonard tube
   e. Snook tube

7. The Bucky grid, which was introduced in 1921, does what?
   a. Improves contrast resolution
   b. Improves spatial resolution
   c. Provides x-ray collimation
   d. Reduces examination time
   e. Reduces patient exposure

8. Which of the following regarding radiation lethality is *true?*
   a. Clarence Dally was the first American to die because of x-ray exposure.
   b. No medical radiation deaths have occurred.
   c. Radiology has always been considered a completely safe occupation.
   d. The first x-ray-induced death did not occur until approximately 1920.
   e. The first x-ray-induced death occurred within a year of Roentgen's discovery.

9. Which of the following describes the Coolidge x-ray tube?
   a. It has a heated cathode.
   b. It has a rotating anode.
   c. It is not as good as the Crookes tube.
   d. It is not in use today.
   e. It was used by Roentgen when he discovered x-rays.

10. Roentgen originally identified x-rays as which of the following?
    a. Alpha rays
    b. Cathode rays
    c. Electrons
    d. X-heat
    e. X-light

11. What are the two simple, general types of x-ray imaging procedures?
    a. Digital and analog
    b. Electromagnetic and ultrasonic
    c. Radiographic and fluoroscopic
    d. Radiographic and tomographic
    e. Roentgenographic and ultrasonic

12. Which of the following provides dynamic x-ray images?
    a. Digital radiography
    b. Doppler ultrasonography
    c. Fluoroscopy
    d. Mammography
    e. Tomography

13. The film base for a radiograph made in 1920 would have been made of which of the following?
    a. Calcium tungstate
    b. Cellulose acetate
    c. Cellulose nitrate
    d. Glass
    e. Tungstate cadmium

14. X-ray beam collimation and filtration do which of the following?
    a. Compromise image quality
    b. Improve spatial resolution
    c. Reduce exposure time
    d. Reduce patient dose
    e. Result in patient discomfort

15. Which of the following imaging modalities was developed *most* recently?
    a. Computed tomography (CT)
    b. Diagnostic ultrasound
    c. Direct digital radiography
    d. Magnetic resonance imaging
    e. Multislice helical CT

16. Which of the following radiation responses was *not* reported before 1910?
    a. Anemia
    b. Death
    c. Epilation
    d. Leukemia
    e. Skin erythema

17. What initial observation led to the discovery of x-rays?
    a. A glow of a plate coated with calcium tungstate located several feet from an energized Coolidge tube in a darkened laboratory.
    b. An exposure on a glass plate coated with photographic emulsion when developed after exposure by a Leonard tube.
    c. Skin damage on the hand of the discoverer.
    d. Skin damage on the hand of the discoverer's wife's hand.
    e. The glow of a plate coated with barium platinocyanide located several feet from an energized Crookes tube.

18. What national certification organization evaluates the proficiency of graduates of educational programs in radiologic technology?
    a. American Association of Physicists in Medicine (AAPM)
    b. American Board of Radiology (ABR)
    c. American Registry of Radiologic Technologists (ARRT)
    d. American Society of Radiologic Technologists (ASRT)
    e. Joint Review Committee on Education in Radiologic Technology (JRCERT)

Worksheet 1-3
Reports of Radiation Injury
Basic Radiation Protection
The Medical Imaging Team

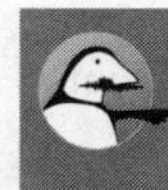

- Radiology is a safe occupation.
- The principal concerns of medical x-ray exposure are cancer and leukemia.
- The occupational dose limit for radiologic technologists is 50 mSv/y (5000 mrem/y).
- Remember the principle of *ALARA*: Maintain radiation exposure *as low as reasonably achievable*.
- The three cardinal principles of radiation protection are: (1) reduce time, (2) increase distance, and (3) use protective shielding where appropriate.
- Radiologic technologists must be certified by the American Registry of Radiologic Technologists; medical physicists must be certified by the American Board of Medical Physics or American Board of Radiology (ABR); interpreting physicians should be certified by the ABR.

EXERCISES

1. One of the cardinal principles of radiation protection states that the radiographer should minimize which of the following?
   a. Distance
   b. kVp
   c. mAs
   d. Shielding
   e. Time

2. Which of the following is *not* included in 10 basic radiation control principles of diagnostic radiology?
   a. Always wear a radiation monitor while at work.
   b. Collimate the x-ray beam to the appropriate field size.
   c. Never stand in the primary beam.
   d. Use high-mA technique.
   e. Wear protective apparel during fluoroscopy.

3. If it is necessary to immobilize a patient during a radiographic examination, the *most* acceptable person to do this is a/an:
   a. 18-year-old brother of the patient
   b. 20-year-old female technologist
   c. 40-year-old male technologist
   d. 50-year-old female friend of the patient
   e. Hospital orderly

4. Which of the following is correctly stated for diagnostic radiology?
   a. Collimation is important only for chest examination.
   b. Copper is used most often as an x-ray filter.
   c. Gonad shields are important for patients of childbearing age.
   d. The radiologic technologist may hold patients for some x-ray examinations.
   e. Radiographic grids reduce patient dose.

5. Which of the following will reduce personnel exposure the *most?*
   a. Collimation of the x-ray beam
   b. Filtration of the x-ray beam
   c. Recording of fluoroscopy time
   d. A high-kVp technique
   e. Use of protective barriers for radiographers

6. When abdominal radiography is conducted on a child, which of the following is *true?*
   a. Gonad shielding is not necessary.
   b. Increasing kVp will increase image contrast.
   c. The parent should hold the child if necessary, and protective apparel should be provided.
   d. The parent should hold the child if necessary, and protective apparel is not necessary.
   e. The technologist should hold the child if necessary.

7. All ***except*** which of the following helps to reduce patient dose?
   a. Cones
   b. Filtration
   c. Gonadal shields
   d. Collimation
   e. Radiographic grids

8. After termination of an x-ray exposure:
   a. No more x-rays are emitted.
   b. The patient continues to emit scatter radiation for a few seconds.
   c. The patient continues to emit scatter radiation for less than 1 second.
   d. The patient is momentarily radioactive.
   e. X-rays continue to be emitted for a few seconds.

9. During fluoroscopy, what should the radiographer always do?
   a. Leave the radiation monitor behind the fixed protective barrier.
   b. Position the radiation monitor under the protective apron.
   c. Remain as close to the patient as possible.
   d. Wear a radiation monitor when examined as a patient.
   e. Wear protective apparel.

10. The main reason for filtering the x-ray beam is to:
   a. Absorb heat
   b. Absorb penetrating x-radiation
   c. Focus the x-ray beam
   d. Reduce patient dose
   e. Sharpen the image

11. Which of the following represents an implementation of a radiation protection procedure?
   a. Avoid repeat examination.
   b. Collimate to the image receptor size.
   c. Avoid abdominal imaging during the first trimester.
   d. Remove filtration.
   e. Wear protective apparel at the control console.

12. Which of the following is an example of an x-ray beam collimator?
   a. Dead-man switch
   b. Elapsed timer
   c. Filter
   d. Positive-beam limitation
   e. Radiographic grid

13. X-ray examination of the pelvis of a woman of reproductive capacity should be limited to which of the following times?
   a. The 10-day interval after the onset of menses
   b. The 10-day interval before the onset of menses
   c. The first 10 days of every month
   d. The last 10 days of every month
   e. There are no restrictions; any time is fine.

14. Which of the following is *true* regarding the discovery of ionizing radiation?
   a. It was predicted by Mendeleev's field theory.
   b. Radioactivity was discovered within a year of Roentgen's discovery.
   c. Roentgen's discovery occurred in 1906.
   d. The apparatus that Roentgen used was called a *Coolidge tube*.
   e. The first radiation fatality occurred in 1920.

15. Generally, x-ray examinations are reserved for which of the following?
   a. Asymptomatic patients
   b. Older patients
   c. Patients who are not pregnant
   d. Symptomatic patients
   e. X-ray personnel

16. Gonad shields should be used:
   a. For all examinations of all patients
   b. On all female patients
   c. On all male patients
   d. When the gonads are in or near the useful beam
   e. When the gonads are in the useful beam

17. Which of the following is the principal reason to avoid repeat examination?
   a. The cost of the procedure is doubled.
   b. The images may be confusing.
   c. The patient is inconvenienced.
   d. The patient receives twice the radiation dose.
   e. The radiographer's workload is doubled.

18. As radiographers, we believe any dose or radiation could be harmful to our patients therefore we follow the _____ principle.
   a. ALARA
   b. BEIR
   c. ICRP
   d. LNT
   e. NCRP

19. Which of the following regarding radiation injury is true?
   a. Clarence Dally was the first American x-ray fatality.
   b. Radiology has always been considered a safe profession.
   c. The first x-ray fatality occurred within a year of the discovery of x-rays.
   d. The first x-ray injury occurred ten years following the discovery of x-rays.
   e. Thomas Edison was the first American x-ray fatality.

20. When present in the examination room during fluoroscopy, what should the radiographer always do?
   a. Leave the radiation monitor behind the fixed protective barrier.
   b. Position the radiation monitor under the protective lead apron.
   c. Position yourself behind the radiologist.
   d. Remain as close to the patient as possible.
   e. Wear protective lead apparel.

Worksheet 1-4
Numeric Prefixes

The numeric prefixes most often encountered in radiology are as follows:

Multiple	Prefix	Symbol
10^{-12}	pico-	p
10^{-9}	nano-	n
10^{-6}	micro-	μ
10^{-3}	milli-	m
10^{-2}	centi-	c
10^{3}	kilo-	k
10^{6}	mega-	M
10^{9}	giga-	G
10^{12}	tera-	T

EXERCISES

1. 10 kilometers (km) is equal to:
   a. 100 m
   b. 1000 m
   c. 10,000 m
   d. 100,000 m
   e. 1,000,000 m

2. A radiographic exposure that lasts $\frac{1}{10}$ s is equal to:
   a. 100 μs
   b. 1 ms
   c. 10 ms
   d. 100 ms
   e. 1000 ms

3. A posteroanterior (PA) chest examination is conducted at 120 kVp. The peak x-ray tube voltage is:
   a. 120 V
   b. 1200 V
   c. 12,000 V
   d. 120,000 V
   e. 1,200,000 V

4. A radiographic exposure made on the 200 mA station is equivalent to:
   a. 2000 μA
   b. 20,000 μA
   c. 200,000 μA
   d. 2,000,000 μA
   e. 20,000,000 μA

5. If you are 160 cm tall, your height is also:
   a. 0.16 m
   b. 16 mm
   c. 16,000 mm
   d. 1.6×10^{6} μm
   e. 1.6×10^{6} nm

6. Which of the following is *correct?*
   a. 1,000,000 eV = 1 keV
   b. 0.001 A = 1 pA
   c. 10^{-7} m = 1 nm
   d. 10 μA = 0.1 mA
   e. $\frac{1}{60}$ s = 17 ms

7. If your mass is 70 kg, it is also:
   a. 0.07 mg
   b. 7000 g
   c. 70,000 g
   d. 7,000,000 mg
   e. 70,000,000 μg

8. Which of the following scientific prefixes is *correct?*
   a. A $\frac{1}{120}$ s exposure is 8 ms.
   b. A 35-keV x-ray has 35×10^{6} eV of energy.
   c. 1 nm is 10^{-12} m.
   d. 1 μBq is 10^{-3} Bq.
   e. 10 kVp is 1000 Vp.

9. A KUB radiograph is made at 82 kVp/200 mA/0.25 s. This is equivalent to:
   a. 0.82×10^{3} kVp/2×10^{-5} μA/2.5×10^{4} ms
   b. 0.82×10^{4} kVp/0.2 A/25 ms
   c. 8.2×10^{6} mVp/2×10^{2} mA/2.5×10^{2} ms
   d. 8.2×10^{7} μVp/2×10^{5} μA/2.5×10^{6} μs
   e. 82×10^{3} Vp/2×10^{-1} A/250 ms

10. The normal source-to-image receptor distance (SID) for an upright chest radiograph is 180 cm. This is equivalent to:
    a. 1.8 m
    b. 18 mm
    c. 180 mm
    d. 1800 μm
    e. 18,000 μm

11. When the radiographic exposure time is ½ s, it is also:
    a. 50 ms
    b. 200 ms
    c. 500 ms
    d. 2000 ms
    e. 5000 ms

12. A fluoroscopic examination is conducted at 1.5 A. This is equivalent to:
    a. 15 mA
    b. 150 mA
    c. 1500 mA
    d. 15,000 mA
    e. 1500 μA

13. The normal x-ray tube potential for a mammogram is 26 kVp. This is equivalent to:
    a. 2.6×10^{-2} Vp
    b. 2.6×10^{-1} Vp
    c. 2.6×10^{2} Vp
    d. 2.6×10^{3} Vp
    e. 2.6×10^{4} Vp

14. The SID for a mobile radiograph is often 90 cm. This is equivalent to:
    a. 9×10^{-2} m
    b. 9×10^{-1} m
    c. 9×10^{0} m
    d. 9×10^{2} m
    e. 9×10^{3} m

15. A radiographic exposure requires 400 ms. This is also:
    a. 0.0004 s
    b. 0.004 s
    c. 0.04 s
    d. 0.4 s
    e. 4 s

16. A radiographic exposure is made at 600 mA, 200 ms. This is equivalent to:
    a. 1.2 mAs
    b. 1.2×10^{1} mAs
    c. 1.2×10^{2} mAs
    d. 1.2×10^{3} mAs
    e. 1.2×10^{4} mAs

17. A chest radiograph is conducted at 125 kVp. This is equivalent to:
    a. 1.25×10^{2} Vp
    b. 1.25×10^{3} Vp
    c. 1.25×10^{4} Vp
    d. 1.25×10^{5} Vp
    e. 1.25×10^{6} Vp

18. An average annual occupational radiation exposure for a radiographer is approximately 5 mSv. This is equivalent to:
    a. 5×10^{-3} Sv
    b. 5×10^{-2} Sv
    c. 5×10^{-1} Sv
    d. 5×10^{0} Sv
    e. 5×10^{2} Sv

19. A lateral chest radiograph will expose a patient to approximately 0.2 mGy_a. This is equivalent to:
    a. 2×10^{1} μGy_a
    b. 2×10^{2} μGy_a
    c. 2×10^{3} μGy_a
    d. 2×10^{4} μGy_a
    e. 2×10^{5} μGy_a

20. The spectrum of visible light extends from approximately 400 to 700 nm. This is equal to:
    a. $(4–7) \times 10^{-4}$ m
    b. $(4–7) \times 10^{-5}$ m
    c. $(4–7) \times 10^{-6}$ m
    d. $(4–7) \times 10^{-7}$ m
    e. $(4–7) \times 10^{-8}$ m

Worksheet 1-5
Radiologic Units

Radiation Exposure:

Air kerma is the kinetic energy transferred from photons to electrons. Air kerma is measured in joules per kilogram (J/kg), where 1 J/kg = 1 Gy_a

1 gray in air (Gy_a) = 1 J/kg (1 roentgen [R] = 2.58 = 10^{-4} coulombs per kilogram [C/kg] of air)

Radiation Absorbed Dose:

Absorbed dose is the radiation energy absorbed per unit mass and has units of J/kg or Gy_t.

1 Gy_t = 1 J/kg = 10^2rad (1 radiation absorbed dose [rad] = 10^2 ergs per gram

[erg/g] = 10^{-2} gray in tissue [Gy_t])

Equivalent Dose:

The sievert is the unit of equivalent dose. It takes into account the effect of different types of radiation.

1 Sv = 1 J/kg = 10^2rem

(1 roentgen equivalent man (rem = 10^2 ergs per gram [erg/g]) = 10^{-2} sieverts [Sv])

Effective Dose:

This measure of radiation intensity accounts for different tissue and organ radiosensitivity. It is used for radiation risk assessment and is expressed in sieverts (Sv); (rem).

Radioactivity:

1 curie (Ci) = 3.7 × 10^{10} atoms disintegrating per second (s^{-1})

3.7 × 1010 becquerel (Bq)

1 Bq = 1 s^{-1}

EXERCISES

1. A radiation monitoring report would express a radiographer's dose equivalent in which of the following?
   a. Becquerel
   b. Curie
   c. Gray
   d. Roentgen
   e. Sievert

2. A posteroanterior chest radiograph delivers approximately what dose to the patient?
   a. 100 eV
   b. 100 J
   c. 100 mR
   d. 100 µGy_a
   e. 100 µGy_t

3. To produce death, mice must be irradiated to a total effective dose of approximately:
   a. 6 eV
   b. 6 Gy_a
   c. 6 Gy_t
   d. 6 J
   e. 6 Sv

4. The approximate output intensity of a radiographic x-ray tube is:
   a. 50 mCi/mAs
   b. 50 mJ/mAs
   c. 50 µGy_a/mAs
   d. 50 µGy_t/mAs
   e. 50 µSv/mAs

5. Tc-99^m is the *most* often used radionuclide in diagnostic nuclear medicine. It is used in quantities of:
   a. MBq
   b. Ci
   c. Gy_a
   d. J
   e. Sv

6. The mGy_a is a unit of measure that specifies which of the following?
   a. Absorption of x-rays
   b. Attenuation of x-rays
   c. Character of x-rays
   d. Intensity of x-rays
   e. Quality of x-rays

7. Which of the following adequately describes the use of the Gy_t?
   a. To measure the energy absorbed by the tissue.
   b. To measure radiation exposure in the air.
   c. To measure the amount of radioactive material.
   d. To measure the occupational exposure received by a radiographer.
   e. To measure the output intensity of an x-ray machine.

8. Which of the following is a classic radiologic unit?
   a. Ampere
   b. Coulomb/kilogram
   c. Joule
   d. rem
   e. Sievert

9. If 20 Gy_t is delivered to 2 g of soft tissue, 1 g of this tissue receives:
   a. 0.5 Gy_t
   b. 10 g-Gy_t
   c. 10 Gy_t
   d. 20 g-Gy_t
   e. 20 Gy_t

10. Absorbed dose can be measured in:
   a. Ergs
   b. Gy
   c. J
   d. keV
   e. kg-Gy

11. Which of the following is *not* a unit of energy?
   a. Calorie
   b. Electron volt
   c. Erg
   d. Gray
   e. Joule

12. Which of the following statements is equivalent?
   a. 1 Gy_t = 1 J/kg
   b. 1 mCi = 37 μC/kg
   c. 1 Sv = 100 erg/g
   d. 200 mrad = 2 cGy
   e. 500 mR = 5 mGy_a

13. Which of the following is a unit of radioactivity?
   a. Bq
   b. Gyt
   c. J
   d. Gya
   e. Sv

14. Absorbed dose can be expressed in:
   a. Bq
   b. Ci
   c. Ergs
   d. eV
   e. J/kg

15. Which of the following demonstrates the proper use of air kerma?
   a. An angiographer receives an occupational exposure of 10 mGy_a.
   b. 100 Gy_t of ^{131}I is administered to image the thyroid.
   c. Patient treatment dose with a linear accelerator unit is 6000 R.
   d. The dose limit for radiologic technologists is 50 mSv/y.
   e. X-ray intensity from a linear accelerator unit is 2 Gy_a/min.

16. In diagnostic radiology, it is acceptable to assume that 1 mGy_a is equal to:
   a. 1 Ci
   b. 1 erg
   c. 1 J
   d. 1 keV
   e. 1 mGy_t

17. In the SI system:
   a. Equivalent dose is expressed in Gy.
   b. kVp is equal to keV.
   c. 1 J is approximately equal to 1 MeV.
   d. 1000 rad is equivalent to 10 Gy.
   e. 1000 rad is equivalent to 100 Sv.

18. Dose rate could be expressed in units of:
   a. Ergs/g
   b. J/kg/min
   c. keV/min
   d. kVp/s
   e. Sv/min

19. When SI is used, radiation exposure is defined in units of coulombs/kilogram. With regard to this unit of measure, which of the following is *true?*
   a. *Coulomb* refers to electrons released in ionization.
   b. *Coulomb* refers to the energy absorbed.
   c. *Kilogram* refers to the mass of radiation.
   d. *Kilogram* refers to the radiation mass.
   e. *Kilogram* refers to the patient's mass.

20. A KUB x-ray examination exposes only a part of the whole body. When accessing the risk of cancer-induction following a KUB, which is most appropriate?
   a. Air kerma
   b. Effective dose
   c. Equivalent dose
   d. Radiation absorbed dose
   e. Tissue dose

21. When applying air kerma, the term kerma stands for ________.
   a. kinetic energy released in mass
   b. kinetic energy released in matter
   c. kinetic energy removed by mass of air
   d. kinetic energy removed by motion artifacts
   e. kinetic effect when removed by motion artifacts

Worksheet 2-1
Standard Units of Measurement

The International System of Units (SI) has been adopted by nearly all countries. It incorporates seven **base units** as its foundation. The base units then are used to develop **derived units**, some of which are identified by **special names**. The radiologic units are examples of derived units with special names.

Seven SI Base Units

Quantity	Name	Symbol
Amount of substance	Mole	mol
Electric current	Ampere	A
Length	Meter	m
Luminous intensity	Candela	cd
Mass	Kilogram	kg
Temperature	Kelvin	K
Time	Second	s

SI-Derived Units With Special Names

Quantity	Name	Symbol	Expression in Terms of Base Units
Electric charge	Coulomb	C	A*s
Electric potential	Volt	V	m*kg/s*A
Energy, work	Joule	J	m*kg/s
Force	Newton	N	m*kg/s
Frequency	Hertz	Hz	1/s
Power	Watt	W	m*kg/s

EXERCISES

1. Which of the following is *not* a base quantity in the SI?
   a. Electric current
   b. Mass
   c. Radiation exposure
   d. Length
   e. Time

2. Which of the following is an SI base unit?
   a. Becquerel
   b. Coulomb
   c. Coulomb/kilogram
   d. Gray
   e. Kilogram

3. Which of the following standards of SI measure is *correct?*
   a. The foot was measured by King Henry VIII.
   b. The meter is related to the visible emission from the Sun.
   c. The meter is the length of an engraved platinum-iridium bar.
   d. The second is based on the rotation of the Earth around the Sun.
   e. The second is based on the vibrations of cesium atoms.

4. Water has a mass density of 1 g/cm^3. Its density is also:
   a. 10^{-3} kg/m^3
   b. 1 kg/m^3
   c. 10 kg/m^3
   d. 10^3 kg/m^3
   e. 10^5 kg/m^3

5. SI stands for which of the following?
   a. Inconsistent system
   b. Incorrect system
   c. Le Système Institutional
   d. Le Système International d'Unités
   e. System International

6. Which of the following is *not* a system of units?
   a. British
   b. CGS
   c. French
   d. MKS
   e. SI

7. Which of the following is an SI name for a base unit?
   a. Celsius
   b. Kilovolt
   c. Milliampere
   d. Newton
   e. Second

8. Which of the following is a unit of energy?
   a. Gray
   b. Joule
   c. Newton
   d. Gram
   e. Sievert
9. Which of the following is expressed in the proper units?
   a. Absorbed dose: Sv
   b. Radioactivity: Gyt
   c. Dose equivalent: mGya
   d. Effective dose: Bq
   e. Exposure: mGy_a
10. Which of the following is an SI-derived unit?
   a. Dyne
   b. Horsepower
   c. Joule
   d. Kelvin
   e. Roentgen
11. Which of the following has units of s^{-1}?
   a. Dose
   b. Exposure
   c. Frequency
   d. Time
   e. Velocity
12. The unit of measure that is the same for all systems of measure is the:
   a. Calorie
   b. Kilogram
   c. Meter
   d. Pound
   e. Second
13. A kilogram is the:
   a. Energy required to raise 1 lb of water 1°C.
   b. Mass of a standard gold bar.
   c. Mass of 1 lb of water.
   d. Mass of $1000 cm^3$ of water.
   e. Temperature rise of 1 lb of water.
14. What unit results when a coulomb is divided by a second?
   a. Ampere
   b. Hertz
   c. Ohm
   d. Gray
   e. Volt
15. What common radiologic unit results from the following? millicoulomb × second =
   a. ESE
   b. kVp
   c. mA
   d. PBL
   e. SID
16. The radiologic unit milliampere-second (mAs) is actually a measure of:
   a. Electric charge
   b. Electric potential
   c. Number of electrons
   d. Potential difference
   e. X-ray intensity
17. Which of the following is a unit of electric potential?
   a. Joule
   b. kVp
   c. mA
   d. mAs
   e. Newton
18. The fundamental unit of force is the:
   a. Coulomb
   b. Joule
   c. Newton
   d. Hertz
   e. Volt

Worksheet 2-2 Newton's Laws

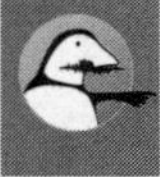

- **Newton's first law**—*Inertia*: When no force is acting on an object, it will continue in its present state of motion or rest.
- **Newton's second law**—*Force*: The force required to change the state of motion of an object is directly proportional to the product of the mass of the object and the acceleration.
- **Newton's third law**—*Reaction*: For every force, there is an equal but opposite force.
- **Mass** is the property of matter that tends to keep a stationary object at rest or that resists a change in the motion of an object that is already moving (Newton's first law).
- **Force** is a push or a pull. Newton's second law, which expresses the concept of force, is his greatest and is represented by the equation:

$$F = ma$$

where

Force (newtons [N]) = Mass (kg) × Acceleration (m/s^2)

- The weight of an object is actually the force of gravitational attraction on its mass. In mathematical terms:

$$W = mg$$

Weight (N) = Mass (kg) × Acceleration (m/s^2)

EXERCISES

1. Which of the following is *not* a correct statement of Newton's laws?
   a. Acceleration is equal to initial velocity plus final velocity, divided by 2.
   b. Force is equal to mass times acceleration.
   c. Momentum is equal to mass times velocity.
   d. Velocity is equal to distance divided by time.
   e. Work is the product of force and distance.

2. Which of the following correctly states Newton's first law of motion?
   a. An object at rest will remain at rest unless acted on by an external force.
   b. An object with mass (m) and acceleration (a) is acted on by a force, given by the equation F = ma.
   c. For every action, there is an opposite and equal reaction.
   d. Matter and energy are related.
   e. The total momentum before any interaction is equal to the total momentum after the interaction.

3. Another name for *velocity* is:
   a. Energy
   b. Mass
   c. Speed
   d. Time
   e. Work

4. When you travel 50 mph, you are also going approximately:
   a. 80 km/h
   b. 100 km/h
   c. 1100 ft/min
   d. 2200 ft/min
   e. 3300 ft/min

5. *Acceleration* is also:
   a. The product of time and distance
   b. The rate of change of time with velocity
   c. The rate of change of velocity with distance
   d. The rate of change of velocity with time
   e. Time squared

6. An automobile travels 30 miles in 30 minutes. Its average velocity is approximately:
   a. 1 mi/min
   b. 33 mi/min
   c. 60 mi/min
   d. 88 mi/min
   e. 99 mi/min

7. The final speed of a dragster in a quarter mile is 80 mph. The average velocity is:
   a. 4 mi/h
   b. 8 mi/h
   c. 16 mi/h
   d. 32 mi/h
   e. 40 mi/h

8. A dragster requires 8 seconds to reach a speed of 80 mph. What is its acceleration?
   a. 1.1 m/s^2
   b. 2.2 m/s^2
   c. 3.3 m/s^2
   d. 4.5 m/s^2
   e. 5.5 m/s^2

9. *Inertia* is:
   a. Mass times acceleration
   b. Newton's second law of motion
   c. Resistance to a change in motion
   d. Velocity divided by time
   e. Velocity times time

10. Which of the following statements refers to a vector quantity?
    a. The car was speeding north at 100 km/h.
    b. The speed of light is 3×10^8 m/s.
    c. The standard man has a mass of 70 kg.
    d. The standard man weighs 70 kg.
    e. The unit of Planck's constant is J-s.

11. A World Series fastball was clocked at 90 mph. How long did that ball take to travel 90 feet to the plate?
    a. Less than 1 s
    b. 1 s
    c. Longer than 2 s
    d. 1.5 s
    e. 2 s

12. How many fundamental laws of motion did Newton formulate?
    a. 1
    b. 2
    c. 3
    d. 4
    e. 5

13. If someone were to fall off the edge of the south rim of the Grand Canyon, the force exerted would be measured in:
    a. kg
    b. J
    c. m/s
    d. mSv
    e. N

14. If the acceleration caused by gravity is 9.8 m/s^2, what is the gravitational force acting on a 50-kg sack pushed off the roof of a 50-story building?
    a. 0.2 N
    b. 5.1 N
    c. 40.2 N
    d. 80 N
    e. 490 N

15. How is momentum *best* described?
    a. For every action, there is an equal and opposite reaction.
    b. It is the force of an object caused by the downward pull of gravity.
    c. It is the product of the mass of an object and its velocity.
    d. It is the relationship between matter and energy.
    e. Objects falling to the Earth accelerate at a constant rate.

16. The total momentum before any interaction is:
    a. An equal and opposite reaction.
    b. Decreased by the property of friction, so it is less after the interaction.
    c. Equal to the total momentum after the interaction.
    d. Greater than the total momentum during the interaction.
    e. Less than the total momentum during the interaction.

17. Which of the following is a unit of work?
    a. Gray
    b. Hertz
    c. Joule
    d. Newton
    e. Watt

18. Which of the following statements about work is *true?*
    a. It can be measured in watts.
    b. It depends on time.
    c. It involves the same units as energy.
    d. It involves time.
    e. It is performed when a large weight is held motionless.

19. When a force is exerted to push a mobile radiographic imaging system, the force would be expressed in what unit?
    a. Joule
    b. Kilogram
    c. Kilovolt
    d. Newton
    e. Gray

Worksheet 2-3 Mechanics

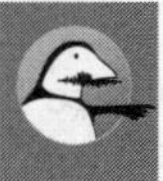

Mechanics is the physics of objects at rest (statics) and objects in motion (dynamics).

WORK

If one exerts a **force** (a push or pull) on a box and moves it across the floor, one does **work** on the box. The following is the formula for work:

$$W = Fd$$

The unit of work is the **joule** (J) if the force is measured in newtons and the distance in meters ($1\,J = 1\,N \times 1\,m$).

ENERGY

A system that is capable of doing work is said to have energy. Energy is the ability to do work, and it can take many forms, including heat energy, electric energy, nuclear energy, and mechanical energy. Mechanical energy may be potential or kinetic:

1. **Potential energy (PE)**: The energy of an object is a result of its position. For example, a brick raised over your head or a coiled spring has PE.
2. **Kinetic energy (KE)**: The energy of an object is a result of its motion.

$$KE = \frac{1}{2} mv^2$$

The basic unit of energy is the **joule**. Other units are also used:

1 electron volt (eV) = 1.6×10^{-19} J
1 erg = 10^{-7} J
1 British thermal unit (BTU) = 1.06 J
1 foot-pound (ft-lb) = 1.36 J
1 kilowatt-hour (kW-h) = 3.6×10^{6} J

POWER

Power is the rate at which work is done. The following is the formula for power:

$$P = W/t$$

The unit of power is the **watt** (1 W = 1 J/s). A commonly used unit of power is the **kilowatt**, which is equal to 1000 W. Another frequently used unit of power is the **horsepower** (hp):

$$1\ hp = 746\ W$$

EXERCISES

1. A radiographer lifts a box onto a platform. The **kinetic energy** of the box depends on _____.
   a. The distance the box is lifted
   b. The force used by the radiographer to lift the box
   c. The mass of the box
   d. The size of the box
   e. The time required to lift the box
2. A radiographer lifts a box onto a platform. The radiographer's **power** output depends on _____.
   a. The distance the box is lifted
   b. The force used by the radiographer to lift the box
   c. The mass of the box
   d. The size of the box
   e. The velocity of the box
3. A radiographer lifts a box onto a platform. The **potential energy** of the box depends on _____.
   a. The force used by the radiographer to lift the box
   b. The mass of the box
   c. The size of the box
   d. The time required to lift the box
   e. The velocity of the box
4. A radiographer lifts a box onto a platform. The total **energy** used depends on _____.
   a. The distance the box is lifted
   b. The force used by the radiographer to lift the box
   c. The size of the box
   d. The time required to lift the box
   e. The velocity of the box
5. A radiographer lifts a box onto a platform. The **work** done depends on _____.
   a. The force used by the radiographer to lift the box
   b. The mass of the box
   c. The size of the box
   d. The time required to lift the box
   e. The velocity of the box
6. Which of the following statements about work is *true?*
   a. It can be measured in watts.
   b. It depends on time.
   c. It has units the same as energy.
   d. It is measured in newtons.
   e. It is performed when a large weight is held motionless.

7. A one-bedroom apartment might use 1000 kW-h of electricity. The kilowatt-hour is a unit of:
   a. Energy
   b. Force
   c. Heat
   d. Potential energy
   e. Power

8. Kinetic energy is directly proportional to:
   a. A vector quantity
   b. Acceleration
   c. Force
   d. Mass
   e. Velocity

9. Which of the following units of energy is *most* fundamental?
   a. Calorie
   b. Electron volt
   c. Erg
   d. Joule
   e. Kilowatt-hour

10. Which of the following is the primary method of heat dissipation from the rotating anode of an x-ray tube?
    a. Conduction
    b. Convection
    c. Convention
    d. Radiation
    e. Reduction

11. Which of the following statements about energy is *true?*
    a. Energy is a force.
    b. Energy is a form of power.
    c. Energy is the ability to do work.
    d. Energy is the rate of doing work.
    e. X-rays can be described by their potential energy.

12. How much work is done in lifting a 1-kg box of film from the floor to a shelf that is 2 m high? (*Hint*: 1 kg = 2.2 lb = 9.8 N)
    a. 1 J
    b. 2.2 J
    c. 4.5 J
    d. 19.6 J
    e. 9 N

13. A car with a 300-hp engine is very fast. The power of the engine is equivalent to how many kilowatts?
    a. 0.4 kW
    b. 2.5 kW
    c. 25 kW
    d. 224 kW
    e. 300 kW

14. Heat is transferred from a glass-enclosed fireplace primarily by:
    a. Conduction
    b. Convection
    c. Convention
    d. Radiation
    e. Temperature

15. A 1-degree change is equal in thermal energy for which two scales?
    a. Absolute and Kelvin
    b. Celsius and absolute
    c. Celsius and Fahrenheit
    d. Celsius and Kelvin
    e. Fahrenheit and Kelvin

16. Which British unit is equivalent to the newton?
    a. Foot-pound
    b. Gram
    c. Joule
    d. Kilogram
    e. Pound

Match the following:

______ 17. Energy	a. Push and pull
______ 18. Force	b. The ability to do work
______ 19. Kinetic energy	c. The energy of motion
______ 20. Power	d. The product of force and distance
______ 21. Work	e. The rate of doing work

Worksheet 3-1 Centuries of Discovery

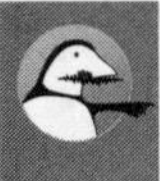

- The concept of an atom has existed through time and developed into the elements of the periodic table.

THE PERIODIC TABLE

- The periodic table is a systematic grouping of elements that is based on the similarity of chemical properties.
- The vertical columns are called **groups**. The horizontal rows are called **periods**.
- As you proceed from left to right in a period, the number of easily removable electrons, called **valence electrons**, increases by one from one group to the next.

EXERCISES

1. Which of the following statements is *true* regarding our understanding of atomic structure?
   a. Rutherford described the nuclear atom.
   b. Rutherford identified cathode rays as particles and constituents of all atoms.
   c. Rutherford is known as the "Father of Radioactivity."
   d. Rutherford is responsible for the periodic table.
   e. Rutherford was an epicurean and envisioned the atom as something familiar to him—plum pudding.

2. In the rendering of the atom by J.J. Thomson:
   a. Electrons were in orbits.
   b. Electrons were distributed throughout the nucleus as plums in a pudding.
   c. Eyes and hooks represented electrons.
   d. He called it the "cathode ray atom."
   e. Uniform positive electrification was theorized.

3. The periodic table presents the elements in the order of:
   a. Atomic charge
   b. Atomic mass
   c. Atomic number
   d. Natural occurrences
   e. Number of isotopes

4. Approximately how many known elements are there?
   a. 50
   b. 100
   c. 150
   d. 200
   e. 300

5. The only element that is *not* placed in any group of the periodic table is:
   a. Helium
   b. Hydrogen
   c. Plutonium
   d. Tungsten
   e. Uranium

6. The horizontal rows in the periodic table are called:
   a. Articles
   b. Compounds
   c. Groups
   d. Molecules
   e. Periods

7. As you move from left to right across the periodic table, what happens to the number of outer-shell electrons from one element to the next?
   a. It decreases by 1.
   b. It decreases by 2.
   c. It increases by 1.
   d. It increases by 2.
   e. It remains constant.

8. Which group in the periodic table contains elements that have only one electron in the outer shell?
   a. Actinide metals
   b. Alkali metals
   c. Halogens
   d. Rare earths
   e. Vapors

9. Which of the following is a transitional element?
   a. Barium
   b. Carbon dioxide
   c. Iodine
   d. Tungsten
   e. Xenon

10. Atoms with all electron shells filled are:
    a. Chemically stable
    b. Chemically very reactive
    c. Found in group 1 of the periodic table
    d. Gases
    e. Radioactive

11. Atoms with three electrons in the outer shell:
    a. Are compounds
    b. Are molecules
    c. Are probably inert gases
    d. Are probably radioactive
    e. Have three valence electrons

12. In the periodic table of the elements, the group number identifies the:
    a. Electron spin state
    b. Number of electrons allowed in the outer shell
    c. Principal quantum number of the outermost shell
    d. Total number of electrons in the atom
    e. Valence state of the atom

13. All of the following are elements *except*:
    a. Carbon
    b. Molybdenum
    c. Oxygen
    d. Steel
    e. Tungsten

14. How many atoms are there in one molecule of sodium bicarbonate ($NaHCO_3$)?
    a. 1
    b. 3
    c. 4
    d. 6
    e. 8

15. Which of the following physicists had a major part in describing the atom as we know it today?
    a. Becquerel
    b. Bohr
    c. Curie
    d. Einstein
    e. Roentgen

16. Which of the following statements is *true?*
    a. A 6000-yd golf course is approximately 10^4 m long.
    b. A football field is approximately 10^3 m long.
    c. An atomic nucleus has a diameter of approximately 10^{-10} m.
    d. In 1 year, light can travel approximately 10^{16} m.
    e. The wavelength of a 100 keV x-ray is approximately 10^{-8} m.

17. The periodic chart of elements is attributed to:
    a. Dimitri Mendeleev
    b. Ernest Rutherford
    c. J.J. Thomson
    d. John Dalton
    e. Niels Bohr

18. Rutherford made what significant contribution to science?
    a. Description of the electron shells
    b. Description of the nuclear atom
    c. Discovery of artificial radioactivity
    d. Discovery of negatively charged electrons
    e. Periodic table of the elements

19. Which of the following statements about atoms is true?
    a. Atomic mass is divided equally between a nucleus and the electrons.
    b. Most of the atom is made up of empty space.
    c. The nucleus is held together by the electrostatic proton-proton attraction.
    d. The number of electrons surrounding the nucleus equals the number of neutrons.
    e. The number of electrons surrounding the nucleus equals the number of protons plus the number of neutrons.

20. Which of the following statements about atoms is true?
    a. Atoms that have the same atomic mass interact the same way chemically.
    b. Atoms that have the same atomic number are atoms of the same element.
    c. Electrons are more tightly bound in little atoms than in big atoms.
    d. M-shell electrons are more tightly bound than L-shell electrons.
    e. Neutron number determines chemical properties.

Worksheet 3-2
Fundamental Particles
Atomic Structure

Matter is composed of atoms. Atoms are composed of fundamental particles called **protons, neutrons**, and **electrons**. The positively charged protons and uncharged neutrons make up the **nucleus** of the atom. The negatively charged electrons revolve around the nucleus in definite orbits, just as the planets orbit the Sun.

The electron is the lightest of the fundamental particles. The mass of the proton is 1836 times larger than the mass of the electron. The neutron mass is 1839 times larger than that of the electron.

The closer electrons are to the nucleus, the more tightly bound they are. The number of electrons in any shell increases to a maximum of $2n^2$, where n is the shell number. No matter how large the atom becomes, however, it normally has the same number of electrons as protons. If this is not the case, the atom is an **ion**.

EXERCISES

1. If $^{129}_{53}I$ is a stable electrically neutral atom, then how many neutrons are there in such an atom?
   a. 53
   b. 76
   c. 129
   d. 182
   e. The question does not give enough information.

2. When oxygen $\left(^{16}_{8}O\right)$ combines with two atoms of hydrogen $\left(^{1}_{1}H\right)$ to form water, the resultant molecule has a total of:
   a. 8 electrons
   b. 10 protons
   c. 16 electrons
   d. 18 protons
   e. 20 nucleons

3. The atomic mass number of an atom is given by the number of:
   a. Electrons
   b. Neutrons
   c. Protons
   d. Protons plus neutrons
   e. Protons plus neutrons plus electrons

4. The atomic number:
   a. Has the symbol "A"
   b. Has the symbol "N"
   c. Is the number of neutrons
   d. Is the number of protons
   e. Is the number of protons plus neutrons

5. Isotopes are atoms:
   a. In the same molecule
   b. Of the same element
   c. That are ions
   d. That contain the same number of neutrons plus protons
   e. With the same number of nucleons

6. Electrons in the M-shell:
   a. Have lower binding energy than those in the N-shell
   b. Never exceed 8 in number
   c. Do not exceed 18 in number
   d. Do not exist in an atom of tungsten (W)
   e. Probably are closer to the nucleus than those in the L-shell

7. $^{12}_{6}C$ and $^{14}_{6}C$ have the same:
   a. A number
   b. N number
   c. Number of neutrons
   d. Number of nucleons
   e. Number of protons

8. The binding energy of an electron to a nucleus:
   a. Increases with increasing distance from the nucleus
   b. Is higher for an L-shell electron than for an M-shell electron
   c. Is higher for a low-Z atom than for a high-Z atom
   d. Is higher for an N-shell than for an M-shell
   e. Depends on the size of an electron

9. How many nucleons does $^{131}_{53}I$ have?
   a. 53
   b. 78
   c. 131
   d. 184
   e. 237

10. The number of protons in the nucleus is called the:
    a. Atomic number
    b. Elemental charge
    c. Ionization state
    d. Mass
    e. Valence

11. A neutron has approximately:
    a. $^{1}/_{2000}$ atomic mass unit (amu) and no charge
    b. 1 amu and no charge
    c. 1 amu and a charge of +1
    d. 4 amu and a charge of +2
    e. 4 amu and no charge

12. How many different types of nucleons are there?
    a. 1
    b. 2
    c. 3
    d. 4
    e. 6

13. Which of the following is a fundamental particle?
    a. Alpha
    b. Beta
    c. Electron
    d. Gamma
    e. Hydrogen

14. Tungsten $^{184}_{74}W$ has how many neutrons?
    a. 74
    b. 110
    c. 184
    d. 258
    e. 332

15. What is the maximum number of electrons permitted in the N-shell?
    a. 8
    b. 18
    c. 24
    d. 32
    e. 50

16. Regarding atomic nomenclature:
    a. Atomic mass is the number of neutrons.
    b. Atomic mass is the number of protons.
    c. Atomic mass is the number of protons minus neutrons.
    d. Atomic mass number determines chemical properties.
    e. Atomic mass number is a whole number.

17. The following atoms are all stable; which has the highest K-shell electron-binding energy?
    a. Al (aluminum)
    b. Hg (mercury)
    c. S (sulfur)
    d. Sr (strontium)
    e. Tc (technetium)

Worksheet 3-3
Atomic Nomenclature
Combinations of Atoms

The atomic mass number and the precise mass of an atom are not the same. Atoms of various elements may combine to form structures called molecules. Quantities of a given molecule are called a chemical compound.

Certain naturally occurring and artificially produced atoms can emit radiation spontaneously. Such atoms are said to be **radioactive**. Radioactivity is the result of instability in the nucleus. Three types of radiation come from the nucleus of a radioactive atom: **alpha (α) particles, beta (β) particles, and gamma (γ) rays.**

- Alpha particles consist of two protons and two neutrons.
- Beta particles are actually electrons that are emitted from the nucleus.
- Gamma rays are the product of electromagnetic radiation of high energy and high penetrability (much like x-rays).

EXERCISES

Match the following.

______ 1. Alpha particle	a.	A particle accelerator used to produce radioisotopes
______ 2. Beta particle	b.	A particle with a charge of -1.602×10^{-19} C
______ 3. Cyclotron	c.	A stable atom that can be made radioactive
______ 4. Gamma ray	d.	A substance composed of atoms with unstable nuclei
______ 5. Gold	e.	An atom that is naturally radioactive
______ 6. Isotope	f.	Atoms with the same number of protons but different numbers of neutrons
______ 7. Radioactive	g.	Radiation that cannot penetrate a sheet of paper material
______ 8. Radioactivity	h.	Spontaneous emission of energy or particles from unstable nuclei
______ 9. Radioisotope	i.	Uncharged radiation; highly penetrating
______ 10. Uranium	j.	Usually produced by particle accelerators from common elements

11. When a radioisotope emits a beta particle:
   a. A gamma ray is always emitted.
   b. A neutron is converted to a proton.
   c. A proton is converted to a neutron.
   d. An electron is converted to a beta particle.
   e. An x-ray is always emitted.

12. Which of the following pairs of atoms are isobars?
   a. ^{129}I and ^{131}I
   b. ^{131}I and ^{198}Hg
   c. ^{2}H and ^{3}H
   d. ^{3}He and ^{3}H
   e. ^{131}I and ^{137}Cs

13. Potassium $\left(^{40}_{19}K\right)$ is a naturally occurring radioisotope that decays by beta emission. Therefore the daughter atom:
   a. Has a mass of approximately 19 amu
   b. Will also be radioactive
   c. Will have 19 neutrons
   d. Will have 40 nucleons
   e. Will have 90 protons

14. Isotopes are:
   a. Atoms that have identical mass and atomic number.
   b. Atoms that have the same atomic mass number but different atomic numbers.
   c. Atoms that have the same atomic number but different atomic mass numbers.
   d. Molecules that consist of identical atoms.
   e. Molecules that have the same number of atoms.

15. The number of disintegrations per second in 2 mCi of ^{99m}Tc is:
   a. 3.7×10^{7}
   b. 3.7×10^{10}
   c. 3.7×10^{12}
   d. 7.4×10^{7}
   e. 7.4×10^{10}

16. With regard to ${}^{90}_{38}Sr^{+2}_{3}$:
    a. The atomic number is 90.
    b. The symbolism indicates that this is a radioactive nuclide.
    c. The valence is 3.
    d. There are 90 neutrons in the nucleus of this atom.
    e. There are a total of 36 electrons in one such atom.

17. Beta emission:
    a. Occurs only with heavy elements
    b. Occurs only with light elements
    c. Occurs only with radioisotopes with long half-lives
    d. Results in the gain of a proton
    e. Results in the loss of 1 amu

18. Alpha emission:
    a. Occurs only with light elements
    b. Occurs only with radioisotopes with long half-lives
    c. Results in the gain of a proton
    d. Results in the loss of 2 amu
    e. Results in the loss of 4 amu

19. After beta emission, the nucleus has:
    a. Decreased in A number by 1
    b. Decreased in Z and A numbers by 1
    c. Decreased in Z number by 1
    d. Increased in A number by 1
    e. Increased in Z number by 1

20. 1 Ci is equivalent to disintegration of how many atoms every second?
    a. 3×10^{8}
    b. 3×10^{10}
    c. 3.7×10^{8}
    d. 3.7×10^{10}
    e. 2.2×10^{12}

21. 10 mCi is equivalent to:
    a. $3.7\ 10^{8}$ Bq
    b. 10^{-6} Ci
    c. 3.7×10^{10} d/s
    d. 10^{-2} nCi
    e. 2.2×10^{12} d/min

22. Which of the following statements about atoms is *true?*
    a. A = Z + N.
    b. A = Z − N.
    c. An alpha emission contains four units of mass and four units of charge.
    d. In a radioactive atom, the number of protons does not equal the number of electrons.
    e. Nucleons are electrons, protons, and neutrons.

23. Which of the following pairs of atoms are isotones?
    a. ${}^{1}_{1}H$ and ${}^{2}_{1}H$
    b. ${}^{130}_{56}Ba$ and ${}^{130}_{56}Ba$
    c. ${}^{130}_{53}I$ and ${}^{131}_{54}Xe$
    d. ${}^{99}Tc$ and ${}^{99m}TC$
    e. ${}^{133}_{54}Xe$ and ${}^{133}_{55}Cs$

24. Isomers are atoms that have different:
    a. Energy states
    b. Filled electron shells
    c. Numbers of neutrons
    d. Numbers of protons
    e. States of ionization

25. Radioisotopes:
    a. Are ionized
    b. Are made with x-rays
    c. Are stable atoms
    d. Have closed electron shells
    e. Have unstable nuclei

26. Which of the following statements about K, a naturally occurring radionuclide deposited in body tissues, is true?
    a. It can be detected by x-rays.
    b. It can be produced by x-rays.
    c. It contributes to our total radiation exposure.
    d. It has 40 electrons.
    e. It has 40 protons.

27. Electrons are:
    a. Arranged in orbits around the nucleus
    b. Composed of neutrons and protons
    c. Organized inside the nucleus
    d. Positively charged
    e. Usually bundled together

Worksheet 3-4 Radioactivity

Radioactivity is due to natural or artificially induced instability in the nucleus of an atom. To become stable, the nucleus decays by emitting alpha, beta, or gamma radiation. Radioactivity is measured in curies or becquerels, preferably becquerels.

$$1 \text{ curie (Ci)} = 3.70 \times 10^{10} \text{ disintegration/s}$$

$$1 \text{ becquerel (Bq)} = 1 \text{ disintegration/s}$$

The quantities of radioactive material used for medical imaging are megabecquerels (MBq) and millicuries (mCi).

$$100 \text{ MBq} = 2.7 \text{ mCi}$$

$$10 \text{ mCi} = 370 \text{ MBq}$$

Radioactivity decreases with time. The time required for the activity of a sample to decay to half of its original value is called the radioactive half-life ($T_{½}$).

EXERCISES

1. Radioactive half-life is the time:
   a. It takes for half of the dose to be delivered
   b. It takes for half of the mass to disappear
   c. It takes for one atom to disintegrate
   d. Required for radioactivity to reach one-half of its original value
   e. When half of the quantity now present remains

2. How many half-lives must elapse before the remaining activity is less than 0.1% of the original activity?
   a. 4 half-lives
   b. 6 half-lives
   c. 8 half-lives
   d. 10 half-lives
   e. 12 half-lives

3. Given a 50 μCi (0.19 MBq) sample of ^{131}I ($T_{½}$ = 8 days), the radioactivity will be 3 μCi after approximately how many days?
   a. 24 days
   b. 32 days
   c. 36 days
   d. 40 days
   e. 44 days

4. A 10 mCi quantity of ^{99m}Tc ($T_{½}$ = 6 hours) is available at 8:00 a.m. At noon on that same day, the radioactivity will be closer to:
   a. 1 mCi than to 3 mCi
   b. 3 mCi than to 5 mCi
   c. 5 mCi than to 8 mCi
   d. 10 mCi than to 8 mCi
   e. 15 mCi than to 10 mCi

5. ^{14}C ($T_{½}$ = 5730 years) is used for archeologic dating. Approximately how old is a tree specimen that contains 3 nCi/g (110 Bq/g) if the original concentration of radioactivity is known to be 12 nCi/g (444 Bq/g)?
   a. 5730 years
   b. Approximately 11,000 years
   c. Approximately 17,000 years
   d. Younger than 5730 years
   e. Older than 17,000 years

6. One hundred mCi (3.7 GBq) of an unknown radionuclide has a half-life of 15 days. Therefore:
   a. 400 mCi should have been available 15 days earlier.
   b. In 15 days, only 25 mCi will remain.
   c. In 1 month, 25 mCi will have decayed.
   d. In 1 month, only 75 mCi will remain.
   e. In 3½ months, the activity will be less than 1 mCi.

7. How much ^{99m}Tc ($T_{½}$ = 6 hours) decays in 24 hours?
   a. 3%
   b. 6%
   c. 14%
   d. 86%
   e. 94%

8. In approximately how many half-lives will the activity of 10 mCi (0.37 GBq) of I ($T_{½}$ = 8 days) be reduced to 0.1 mCi (3.7 MBq)?
   a. 3.3 half-lives
   b. 10 half-lives
   c. 12.5 half-lives
   d. 50 half-lives
   e. 100 half-lives

9. Which of the following statements about a given radioisotope is *true?*
   a. As the number of atoms decreases, the half-life decreases.
   b. The half-life increases as the decay constant increases.
   c. The number of radioactive atoms decreases linearly with time.
   d. The percentage of atoms decaying per unit of time decreases.
   e. The percentage of atoms decaying per unit of time is constant.

10. If the half-life of $^{131}_{53}I$ is 8 days, approximately how much $^{131}_{53}I$ remains of an original shipment of 50 μCi (1.9 MBq) after 24 days?
   a. 25 nCi
   b. 25 nCi
   c. 3 μCi
   d. 6 μCi
   e. 12 μCi

11. 10 mCi of ^{99m}Tc is a normal patient dose for imaging. How many becquerels is this?
   a. 2.2×10^8 Bq
   b. 3.7×10^8 Bq
   c. 2.2×10^{11} Bq
   d. 3.7×10^{11} Bq
   e. 3.7×10^{12} Bq

12. $^{131}_{53}I$ has a half-life of 13 hours. If 150 μCi (5.7 MBq) is available at noon on Wednesday, approximately how much will remain at 5:00 p.m. on Friday?
   a. 10 μCi
   b. 20 μCi
   c. 30 μCi
   d. 40 μCi
   e. 50 μCi

13. An unknown radioisotope is assayed to be 40 μCi (15 MBq) at 9:00 a.m. on Monday. An assay at 9:00 p.m. on Tuesday yields a result in 2.5 μCi (0.1 MBq). What is the half-life of the radioisotope?
   a. 3 hours
   b. 6 hours
   c. 9 hours
   d. 12 hours
   e. 18 hours

14. Use the following graph to estimate the percentage of radioactivity that remains after 2½ half-lives.

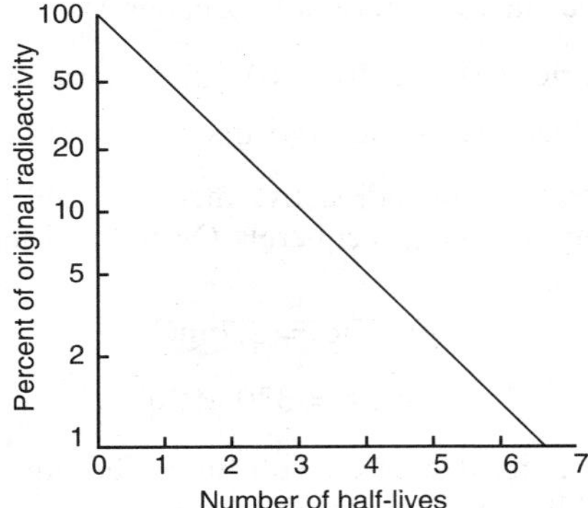

   a. 2½%
   b. 5%
   c. 16%
   d. 50%
   e. 75%

15. The shape of the radioactive decay curve is:
   a. A concave-down curve on linear paper
   b. A concave-up curve on semi-log paper
   c. A straight line on linear paper
   d. A straight line on semi-log paper
   e. Linear and nonthreshold

Worksheet 3-5
Types of Ionizing Radiation

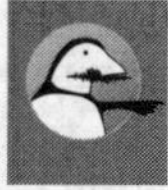

- Radiation is the transfer of energy from one position or medium to another.
- There are two types of radiation: ionizing and nonionizing.
- There are two sources of radiation: naturally occurring radiation and man-made radiation.
- Ionizing radiation is any radiation that can remove an orbital electron from an atom.
- There are two types of ionizing radiation: particulate and electromagnetic.

I. Particulate
   a. Alpha (α) particles
   b. Beta (β) particles
   c. Other nuclear particles

II. Electromagnetic
   a. Gamma (γ) rays
   b. X-rays

EXERCISES

1. The difference between electrons and beta particles is:
   a. Beta particles are ionizing.
   b. Beta particles have higher energy.
   c. Electrons have higher mass.
   d. Electrons have higher velocities.
   e. Their origin.

2. In the air:
   a. A gamma ray does not normally travel farther than 10 m.
   b. Alpha particles have a range of 1 to 10 cm.
   c. Alpha particles travel farthest.
   d. An x-ray does not normally travel farther than 1 m.
   e. Beta particles have a range of 1 to 10 mm.

3. The amount of energy acquired when an electron is accelerated by a potential difference of 1 V is:
   a. 1 Ci
   b. 1 eV
   c. 1 J
   d. 1 mGy_a
   e. 1 mGy_t

4. Alpha particles:
   a. Are similar to hydrogen nuclei
   b. Are useful in nuclear medicine
   c. Contain two electrons
   d. Have an A number of 4
   e. Have a Z number of 4

5. Of the following radiations, the *most* penetrating is a:
   a. 10 keV x-ray
   b. 100 keV gamma ray
   c. 0.01 MeV x-ray
   d. 2.1 MeV beta particle
   e. 4.8 MeV alpha particle

6. The difference between x-rays and gamma rays is:
   a. Gamma rays always have higher energy than x-rays.
   b. Gamma rays have higher mass.
   c. Gamma rays travel faster.
   d. Their origin.
   e. X-rays produce bremsstrahlung radiation and gamma rays do not.

7. X-rays have:
   a. 1 amu and are neutral
   b. A negative charge and no rest mass
   c. No mass and a charge of −1
   d. No mass and a charge of +2
   e. No mass and no charge

8. Given the general characteristics of ionizing radiation:
   a. All photons travel in straight lines, even in the presence of a magnetic field.
   b. As x-ray energy increases, so does linear energy transfer (LET).
   c. The neutron is a chargeless particle and is therefore nonionizing radiation.
   d. The range of a beta particle in tissue can extend to a depth of 10 cm.
   e. The range of gamma rays in air normally does not exceed 1 m.

9. Which of the following types of radiation are emitted from outside the nucleus?
   a. Alpha particles
   b. Beta particles
   c. Gamma rays
   d. Neutrinos
   e. X-rays

10. As compared with particulate radiation, electromagnetic radiation:
    a. Has a higher electrostatic charge
    b. Has higher LET
    c. Is heavier
    d. Is more densely ionizing
    e. Is more penetrating

11. When electromagnetic radiation is compared with particulate radiation, it is *true* that:
    a. Both interact by ionization and excitation.
    b. Particulate radiation exists only at the speed of light.
    c. They are equally penetrating.
    d. They have equal mass.
    e. They have nearly equal LET.

12. Particulate ionizing radiation:
    a. Can include any type of subatomic particle
    b. Has greater range than electromagnetic radiation
    c. Includes ultrasound
    d. Travels at the speed of light
    e. Usually has low LET

13. Electromagnetic ionizing radiation:
    a. Comes from both inside and outside the nucleus
    b. Has a lower velocity than light
    c. Has a lower velocity than particulate radiation
    d. Includes alpha and beta particles
    e. Includes therapeutic ultrasound

14. X-rays and gamma rays are examples of electromagnetic radiation. In addition, they both have:
    a. No electrostatic charge
    b. Small mass
    c. The same origin
    d. The velocity of ultrasound
    e. Variable velocity

15. Which of the following is an example of ionizing radiation?
    a. Energetic protons
    b. Microwaves
    c. MRI
    d. Therapeutic ultrasound
    e. Ultraviolet radiation

16. How does the energy of a gamma ray compare with the energy of an x-ray?
    a. The question does not give enough information.
    b. They are equal.
    c. The energy of gamma rays is greater than the energy of x-rays.
    d. The energy of gamma rays is less than the energy of x-rays.
    e. The energy of gamma rays is much greater than the energy of x-rays.

17. What are the two principal classes of ionizing radiation?
    a. Diagnostic and particulate
    b. MRI and electromagnetic
    c. MRI and ultrasound
    d. Particulate and electromagnetic
    e. Particulate and ultrasound

18. Which of the following is *not* ionizing radiation?
    a. Auger electrons
    b. Beta particles
    c. Neutrons
    d. Therapeutic ultrasound
    e. X-rays

Worksheet 4-1 Photons

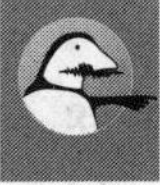

An x-ray photon is a quantum of electromagnetic energy.

The wave equation is as follows:

$v = \lambda \times f$ for velocity = wavelenth × frequency

Electromagnetic radiation always travels at the speed of light (3×10^8 m/s), so $v = c$ and, for electromagnetic radiation, $c = \lambda \times f$. The unit of frequency is the hertz (1 Hz = 1 cycle per second).

At a given velocity, wavelength and frequency are inversely proportional.

EXERCISES

1. X-ray wavelength is:
   a. Directly proportional to frequency
   b. Directly proportional to velocity
   c. Inversely proportional to frequency
   d. Inversely proportional to velocity
   e. Usually designated by "c"

2. Which of the following is *true* for both a 100 keV x-ray and a 10 keV gamma ray?
   a. They have equal frequencies.
   b. They have equal negative charges.
   c. They have equal wavelengths.
   d. They have the same origin.
   e. They have zero mass.

3. A frequency of 1 MHz is:
   a. 1 cycle/s
   b. 10^2 cycles/s
   c. 10^3 cycles/s
   d. 10^6 cycles/s
   e. 10^9 cycles/s

4. When the frequency of electromagnetic radiation is increased 10-fold:
   a. The velocity decreases to ⅒.
   b. The velocity increases 10 times.
   c. The wavelength remains constant.
   d. The wavelength decreases to ⅒.
   e. The wavelength increases 10 times.

5. A single unit of electromagnetic radiation is also called a/an:
   a. Ion
   b. Photon
   c. Proton
   d. Quark
   e. Strange

6. Light has a constant velocity of $c = 3 \times 10^8$ m/s. Therefore:
   a. Its energy increases with increasing wavelength.
   b. Its frequency decreases with increasing wavelength.
   c. Its mass increases with increasing frequency.
   d. Its velocity is also 3×10^{12} cm/s.
   e. Its velocity is also 3×10^{12} mm/s.

7. The frequency of electromagnetic radiation is:
   a. Measured in disintegrations per second
   b. Measured in hertz
   c. Measured in meters per second
   d. Proportional to the wavelength
   e. Proportional to velocity

8. When one uses the sine wave as a model:
   a. Amplitude and frequency are directly proportional.
   b. Amplitude and wavelength are directly proportional.
   c. The distance from one peak to the next is the wavelength.
   d. The distance from one valley to the next is the frequency.
   e. The energy is proportional to amplitude.

9. Given the sine wave model of electromagnetic radiation:
   a. Amplitude and velocity are inversely related.
   b. Frequency and velocity are inversely related.
   c. Frequency times amplitude is a constant.
   d. Frequency times velocity is a constant.
   e. Frequency times wavelength is a constant.

10. Which of the following has a constant value for all electromagnetic radiation?
    a. Frequency
    b. Mass
    c. Origin
    d. Velocity
    e. Wavelength
11. The velocity of light is:
    a. 3×10^8 cm/s
    b. 3×10^{10} cm/s
    c. 3×10^{12} cm/s
    d. 3.7×10^{10} m/s
    e. 3.7×10^8 m/s
12. The amplitude of a sine wave is its:
    a. Frequency
    b. Minimum to maximum
    c. Velocity
    d. Wavelength
    e. Zero to maximum
13. The frequency of a sine wave is:
    a. The distance from crest to crest
    b. The distance from crest to valley
    c. The minimum to maximum
    d. The number of seconds that pass per crest
    e. The number of valleys that pass per second
14. The wave equation is described as follows:
    a. The product of frequency and velocity is constant.
    b. Velocity is frequency divided by wavelength.
    c. Velocity is wavelength divided by frequency.
    d. Wavelength is the product of velocity and frequency.
    e. Wavelength is velocity divided by frequency.
15. The velocity of ultrasound in tissue is 1540 m/s. If a 1 MHz transducer is used, what will be the wavelength of the ultrasound?
    a. 15.4 μm
    b. 1.54 mm
    c. 1540 mm
    d. 15.4 cm
    e. 1540 m
16. A 1 tesla magnetic resonance imaging device operates at a radiofrequency of 42 MHz. What is the wavelength of this radiation?
    a. 4.2 mm
    b. 7.1 mm
    c. 42 cm
    d. 7.1 m
    e. 42 m

If the figure below represents a wave traveling at 25 cm/s, compute the following:

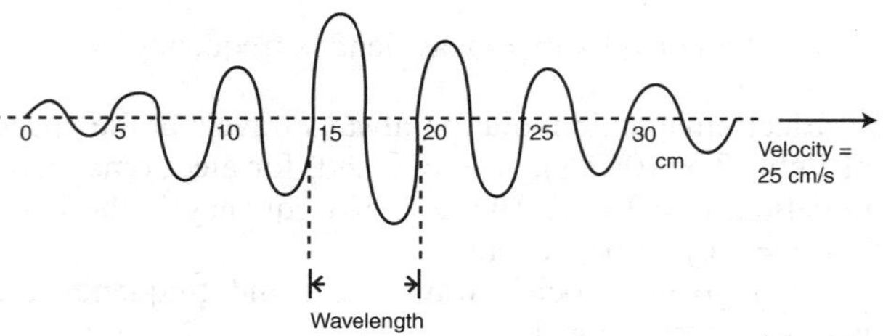

17. How many cycles occur in 1 s (frequency)?
    a. 1
    b. 2
    c. 3
    d. 4
    e. 5
18. How much time is necessary for two cycles?
    a. 0.1 s
    b. 0.2 s
    c. 0.3 s
    d. 0.4 s
    e. 0.8 s
19. What is the wavelength?
    a. 5 cm
    b. 10 cm
    c. 15 cm
    d. 20 cm
    e. 25 cm

Worksheet 4-2 Electromagnetic Spectrum

The electromagnetic (EM) spectrum includes many types of EM radiation that extend over 35 orders of magnitude from low-energy radio waves to high-energy x-rays and y-rays. Each region of the EM spectrum can be identified by energy, wavelength, or frequency through the following equations:

$$E = hf = hc/\lambda \text{ and } c = \lambda f$$

Traditionally, x-rays are identified by their energy, visible light by its wavelength, and radio waves by their frequency.

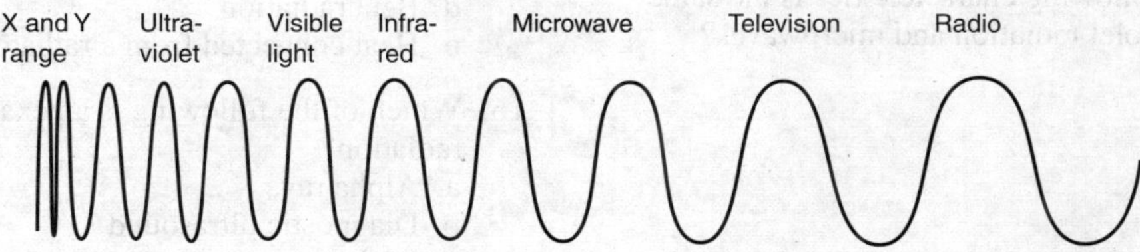

EXERCISES

1. A photon that has energy of approximately 1 eV is *most* likely:
   a. A gamma ray
   b. A radio emission
   c. An x-ray
   d. Therapeutic ultrasound
   e. Visible light

2. When the EM spectrum is considered, photons of a radio broadcast have relatively:
   a. High energy and long wavelengths
   b. High energy and short wavelengths
   c. High frequency and low energy
   d. Low energy and long wavelengths
   e. Low energy and short wavelengths

3. When white light is refracted through a prism, the following colors are emitted. Which has the longest wavelength?
   a. Blue
   b. Orange
   c. Red
   d. Ultraviolet
   e. Yellow

4. Invisible photons on the long-wavelength side of the visible-light spectrum can create a problem in the darkroom. Which of the following types of light are these photons likely to be?
   a. Green light
   b. Infrared light
   c. Laser light
   d. Maser light
   e. Ultraviolet light

5. The principal difference between x-rays and gamma rays is their:
   a. Energy
   b. Frequency
   c. Origin
   d. Velocity
   e. Wavelength

6. Radiation emitted from a standard radio broadcast antenna:
   a. Has a higher frequency than gamma rays
   b. Has a higher frequency than microwaves
   c. Has relatively high energy
   d. Is EM radiation
   e. Is sound

7. For any EM radiation:
   a. An increase in frequency results in an increase in energy.
   b. An increase in velocity results in an increase in energy.
   c. An increase in velocity results in an increase in frequency.
   d. An increase in wavelength results in an increase in energy.
   e. An increase in wavelength results in higher frequency.

8. EM radiation:
   a. Exists at zero velocity
   b. Exists only if its velocity is 3×10^8 m/s
   c. Has energy represented by amplitude
   d. Has mass that increases with increasing velocity
   e. Is usually shown as a square wave

9. If an x-ray imaging system is operated at 40 kVp, then:
   a. 20 keV x-rays are emitted.
   b. All x-rays are emitted at 40 keV.
   c. Non-ionizing x-rays are emitted.
   d. X-rays up to 80 keV are emitted.
   e. Zero-energy x-rays are emitted.

10. A photon of red light:
    a. Comes from a nucleus
    b. Has a higher frequency than an x-ray
    c. Has a longer wavelength than a photon of green light
    d. Has more energy than blue light
    e. Has the same energy as microwaves

11. Which of the following characteristics is the same for both ultraviolet radiation and microwaves?
    a. Amplitude
    b. Energy
    c. Frequency
    d. Velocity
    e. Wavelength

12. Visible light cannot be:
    a. Absorbed
    b. Diffracted
    c. Reflected
    d. Refracted
    e. Weighed

13. X-rays can be:
    a. Attenuated
    b. Compacted
    c. Ionized
    d. Subdivided
    e. Weighed

14. The EM spectrum includes:
    a. Particulate radiation at the speed of light
    b. Radiation described by the following formula: Wavelength = Frequency × Velocity
    c. Radiation with physical properties determined by mass
    d. X-rays and radar with the speed of light in a vacuum
    e. X-rays, gamma rays, electrons, and neutrons that are used in medicine

15. Which of the following types of radiation would be classified as EM?
    a. 5 MHz therapeutic ultrasound
    b. 30 m radio broadcast
    c. 1000 Hz sound
    d. Beta radiation
    e. Heat convected from a radiator

16. Which of the following is an example of EM radiation?
    a. Alpha rays
    b. Diagnostic ultrasound
    c. Positrons
    d. Protons
    e. Ultraviolet light

17. Examples of EM radiation would *not* include:
    a. 1.5 T, 63 MHz MRI
    b. Cell phone signals
    c. Forced-air heat
    d. Light from an exit sign
    e. Phosphorescence from a watch dial

18. Which of the following is *not* an example of EM radiation?
    a. Gamma rays
    b. Grenz rays
    c. Laser radiation
    d. Starlight
    e. Ultrasonic diathermy

Worksheet 4-3 Wave-Particle Duality

E = hf (quantum mechanics)

$$E = hf$$

where E = energy in joules, h = 6.63×10^{-34} J-s, f represents frequency, and h is the Planck constant. $E = mc^2$ (relativity).

$$E = mc^2$$

where E = energy in joules and c = 3×10^8 m/s, the velocity of an x-ray.

To understand the true nature of photon radiation, both wave and particle concepts must be retained because wavelike properties are exhibited in some experiments and particle-like properties are exhibited in others.

Photons interact with matter most easily when the matter is approximately the same size as the photon wavelength. X-rays behave as though they are particles. Visible light and radio-television emission behaves as a wave.

EXERCISES

1. Which of the following is *not* a characteristic of the wave model of radiation?
   a. Collision
   b. Diffraction
   c. Reflection
   d. Refraction
   e. Transmission

2. Which of the following *most* closely represents the term *attenuation?*
   a. Absorption of x-rays
   b. Deflection of x-rays
   c. Light absorbed in black glass
   d. Light reflected from a mirror
   e. Light transmitted through frosted glass

3. When a radiograph is viewed, one might properly state that:
   a. Bony structures are radiolucent.
   b. Fat is radiopaque.
   c. Fat is radioreflective.
   d. Lung tissue is radiolucent.
   e. Soft tissue is radiopaque.

4. The development of modern quantum mechanics is attributed to:
   a. Albert Nobel
   b. Ernest Rutherford
   c. Max Planck
   d. Niels Bohr
   e. William Coolidge

5. According to quantum mechanics, the energy of an x-ray is:
   a. Dependent on its origin
   b. Dependent on its velocity
   c. Directly proportional to its wavelength
   d. Inversely proportional to its wavelength
   e. Proportional to its amplitude

6. The expression that relates x-ray energy and wavelength through Planck's constant is:
   a. $E = hf$
   b. $E = hc$
   c. $E = hc/\lambda$
   d. $E = h/c\lambda$
   e. $E = \lambda c/h$

7. Which of the following statements about visible light is *true?*
   a. It can travel with any velocity up to 3×10^8 m/s.
   b. It is deflected by a magnetic field.
   c. It sometimes behaves like a wave.
   d. Its energy is directly proportional to its wavelength.
   e. The photoelectric effect demonstrates the wave model.

8. Visible light:
   a. Consists of short-wavelength red radiation and long-wavelength blue radiation
   b. Has a higher frequency than ultraviolet light
   c. Has a shorter wavelength than microwaves
   d. Has a wavelength range of 1 to 100 mm
   e. Interacts with matter in the same way that x-rays do

9. Which of the following terms is *not* associated with visible-light interaction?
   a. Absorption
   b. Reflection
   c. Refraction
   d. Transmission
   e. Vaporization

10. Which statement about visible light is *correct?*
    a. Black glass is lucent.
    b. If matter absorbs visible light, it is transparent.
    c. If matter attenuates visible light, it is opaque.
    d. If visible light is transmitted but attenuated, the matter is transparent.
    e. If visible light is transmitted unattenuated, the matter is lucent.

11. In radiographs of bony structures embedded in soft tissue, the bone is:
    a. Radiolucent
    b. Radiopaque
    c. Radiorefracted
    d. Translucent
    e. Transopaque

12. Which of the following statements about photon interaction is *true?*
    a. Air is transparent and radiopaque.
    b. Frosted glass is transparent.
    c. Lead is radiopaque.
    d. Soft tissue is radiopaque.
    e. Window glass is opaque.

13. Which type of electromagnetic radiation is *not* used for medical imaging?
    a. Gamma rays
    b. Microwaves
    c. Radiofrequency
    d. Visible light
    e. X-rays

14. When compared with visible light, x-rays have greater:
    a. Charge
    b. Frequency
    c. Mass
    d. Velocity
    e. Wavelength

15. Which of the following types of electromagnetic radiation interacts with matter such as a particle?
    a. Gamma rays
    b. Infrared radiation
    c. Microwaves
    d. Radio frequencies

16. At what level should visible light interact *most* readily?
    a. Atomic
    b. Molecular
    c. Nucleon
    d. Organ
    e. Tissue

17. Compared with red light, green light has greater:
    a. Charge
    b. Energy
    c. Mass
    d. Velocity
    e. Wavelength

18. The equivalent mass of an x-ray may be computed using:
    a. $m = hc/\lambda$
    b. $m = hc/f$
    c. $m = h\lambda/c^2$
    d. $m = hf/c^2$
    e. $m = hf\lambda/c^2$

19. A surface of which color reflects the *most* light?
    a. Black
    b. Blue
    c. Green
    d. Red
    e. White

Worksheet 4-4
Inverse Square Law

Radiation intensity decreases rapidly as the distance from the source increases. The intensity of radiation is inversely proportional to the square of the distance from the source to the object.

Inverse square law:

$$I_1 / I_2 = d_2^2/d_1^2 = (d_2/d_1)^2$$

where I_1 is the intensity at distance d_1 from the source, and I_2 is the intensity at distance d_2 from the source.

EXERCISES

1. A source of ^{99m}Tc produces a radiation intensity of 1.5 μGy_a/h (150 mR/h) at 10 m. At what distance does the exposure rate equal 10 μGy_a/h?
   a. 3.3 m
   b. 3.9 m
   c. 5.0 m
   d. 6.7 m
   e. 8.2 m

2. If the exposure rate of 1 m from a source is 9 mR/h (90 μGy_a/h), what is the exposure rate of 3 m from the source?
   a. 90 μGy_a /h
   b. 30 μGy_a /h
   c. 10 μGy_a /h
   d. 9 μGy_a /h
   e. 1 μGy_a /h

3. The inverse square law states that:
   a. Intensity and distance are proportional.
   b. Intensity is directly proportional to the square of the distance.
   c. Intensity is inversely proportional to the square of the distance.
   d. The square of the intensity is directly proportional to the distance.
   e. The square of the intensity is inversely proportional to the distance.

4. The inverse square law is a result of:
   a. Absorption
   b. Attenuation
   c. Divergence
   d. Scatter
   e. Transmission

5. The inverse square relationship applies to which of the following sources?
   a. Gamma ray
   b. Plane
   c. Point
   d. Ultrasound
   e. X-ray

6. Which of the following emissions is likely to obey the inverse square law?
   a. Heat from an iron skillet
   b. Infrared radiation from a patient
   c. Skylight
   d. Visible light from a 2-m fluorescent bulb
   e. X-rays from a mobile imaging system

7. To apply the inverse square law, one must know:
   a. Energy, distance, and intensity
   b. One distance and one intensity
   c. The frequency or the wavelength of radiation
   d. Two distances and one intensity
   e. Two intensities and two distances

8. If the distance from a point source is tripled, the intensity will be:
   a. Nine times
   b. One-half
   c. One-ninth
   d. One-third
   e. Three times

9. If an instrument positioned 1 m from a point source is moved 50 cm closer to the source, the radiation intensity will:
   a. Decrease by a factor of 2
   b. Decrease by a factor of 4
   c. Increase by a factor of 2
   d. Increase by a factor of 4
   e. Remain constant

10. The distance from the Earth to the Sun is approximately 150 million km. If the Earth were orbiting the Sun at 50 million km, the solar intensity on the surface of the Earth would be:
    a. 3 times more intense
    b. 9 times more intense
    c. 12 times more intense
    d. 27 times more intense
    e. The same

11. A linear source of radium is 15 mm long. Such a source of radiation obeys the inverse square law at approximately what minimum distance from the source?
   a. At contact
   b. 15 mm
   c. 25 mm
   d. 75 mm
   e. 105 mm

12. How far from a 1-m fluorescent bulb must one be before its light approximately obeys the inverse square law?
   a. 1 m
   b. 2 m
   c. 3 m
   d. 5 m
   e. 7 m

13. A ^{137}Cs source used for instrument calibration has an intensity of 1 mGy_a/h (100 mR/h) at 20 cm. What would the intensity be 40 cm from the source?
   a. 0.08 mGy_a/h
   b. 0.12 mGy_a/h
   c. 0.25 mGy_a/h
   d. 0.5 mGy_a/h
   e. 0.75 mGy_a/h

14. The exposure rate from a ^{60}Co source used in radiation therapy is 1 Gy_a/min (100 R/min) at 80 cm. What would the exposure rate be 40 cm from the source?
   a. 0.25 Gy_a/min
   b. 0.50 Gy_a/min
   c. 1.0 Gy_a/min
   d. 2.0 Gy_a/min
   e. 4.0 Gy_a/min

15. A radiographic technique produces a patient dose of 2 mGy_a (200 mrad) at a source-to-skin distance (SSD) of 80 cm. What would be the patient dose at an SSD of 160 cm if the technique remains the same?
   a. 0.5 mGy_a
   b. 0.8 mGy_a
   c. 1.0 mGy_a
   d. 2.0 mGy_a
   e. 4.0 mGy_a

16. A radiographic technique produces an exposure of 2 mGy_a (200 mR) at a source-to-image receptor distance (SID) of 100 cm. What would the exposure be at an SID of 180 cm?
   a. 0.31 mGy_a
   b. 0.55 mGy_a
   c. 0.62 mGy_a
   d. 1.11 mGy_a
   e. 1.25 mGy_a

17. A radiograph produced at a SID of 100 cm results in an exposure of 1 mGy_a (100 mR). What would be the exposure if the SID were reduced to 90 cm?
   a. 0.72 mGy_a
   b. 0.81 mGy_a
   c. 0.90 mGy_a
   d. 1.11 mGy_a
   e. 1.23 mGy_a

Worksheet 4-5 X-Ray Photons

X-rays also may be thought of as bundles of energy called *quanta* or *photons*. These x-ray photons travel at the speed of light, have direction, possess no mass or charge, and have electric and magnetic components that vary in a sinusoidal fashion. X-rays adhere to the following mathematical relationships:

$$c = \lambda \qquad E = mc^2$$

$$E = hf \qquad \lambda(\text{nm}) = \frac{1.24}{\text{keV}}$$

$$E = \frac{hc}{\lambda}$$

EXERCISES

1. Which of the following terms is associated with diagnostic imaging?
   a. Diffraction x-rays
   b. Grenz x-rays
   c. Megavoltage x-rays
   d. Superficial x-rays
   e. Supervoltage x-rays

2. Which of the following terms does *not* apply to an x-ray?
   a. Absorption
   b. Attenuation
   c. Diffraction
   d. Penetration
   e. Reflection

3. Given two x-rays, one of 50 keV and the other of 70 keV, the 70 keV x-ray:
   a. Is most likely radioactive
   b. Most likely came from a nucleus
   c. Has a higher velocity
   d. Has a longer wavelength
   e. Has a higher frequency

4. In the normal representation of an x-ray:
   a. Energy is amplitude.
   b. Mass is indicated by *c*.
   c. Velocity is the speed of light.
   d. Velocity varies from zero to the speed of light.
   e. Wavelength changes from short to long and back to short again.

5. The energy of an x-ray photon is directly proportional to its:
   a. Frequency
   b. Mass
   c. Velocity
   d. Velocity squared
   e. Wavelength

6. In a vacuum, x-rays travel with a velocity of:
   a. 186,000 km/hr
   b. 186,000 mph
   c. 3×10^{10} m/s
   d. 3×10^{10} cm/s
   e. 3.7×10^{10} cm/s

7. Which of the following is greater for a 30 keV x-ray than for a 60 keV x-ray?
   a. Charge
   b. Frequency
   c. Mass
   d. Velocity
   e. Wavelength

8. Which of the following electromagnetic radiations is in the diagnostic x-ray region?
   a. 78 eV
   b. 12,000 eV
   c. 65 keV
   d. 36 MeV
   e. 14 meV

9. The photon energy of an x-ray whose wavelength is 10 nm may be obtained *most* easily from which of the following?
   a. $E = mc^2$
   b. $E = hf$
   c. $E = hc/\lambda$
   d. $E = \lambda n$
   e. $E = \lambda/hc$

10. When x-rays are described, it can be said that:
    a. They are deflected by a very strong magnet.
    b. They can combine with other x-rays to form an atom.
    c. They can create molecules.
    d. They have a longer wavelength than radio waves.
    e. They travel in straight lines.

11. X-ray photons:
    a. Are part of the ultrasonic spectrum
    b. Are relatively long-wavelength electromagnetic radiation
    c. Have a higher frequency than visible light
    d. Have a longer wavelength than radio frequencies
    e. Have the same velocity as ultrasound

12. The energy of an x-ray:
    a. Can be computed from its mass
    b. Depends on its charge
    c. Increases with increasing wavelength
    d. Is a function of the Einstein constant
    e. Is inversely proportional to its wavelength

13. The model used to describe an x-ray photon:
    a. Consists of an S wave
    b. Has a radiofrequency field and a visual field
    c. Has an electric field and an ultrasonic field
    d. Has an ultrasonic field and a magnetic field
    e. Is a sine wave

14. The Planck constant has units of:
    a. J
    b. J-eV
    c. J-kg
    d. J-s
    e. N-s

15. Which of the following characteristics is the same for both x-ray photons and light photons?
    a. Amplitude
    b. Energy
    c. Frequency
    d. Velocity
    e. Wavelength

16. X-rays:
    a. Have a mass of 1 amu and are neutral
    b. Have a negative charge and zero rest mass
    c. Have a positive charge and zero rest mass
    d. Have zero rest mass and a charge of plus two
    e. Have zero rest mass and are neutral

17. In the model of an x-ray:
    a. The amplitude of the sine wave is related to its energy.
    b. The frequency of the sine wave is related to its velocity.
    c. The wavelength of the sine wave is related to its velocity.
    d. Two sine waves are positioned perpendicular to each other.
    e. Two sine waves are superimposed.

18. Diagnostic x-rays are:
    a. High-energy electromagnetic radiation
    b. Long-wavelength electromagnetic radiation
    c. Observed with varying velocity
    d. Photons with intermediate mass
    e. Photons with low frequency

19. An x-ray also can be correctly called a:
    a. Mass
    b. Photon
    c. Pronon
    d. Proton
    e. Quantity

Worksheet 4-6 Matter and Energy

Matter (mass) is defined by its energy equivalence. Einstein expressed the equivalence of mass and energy with the following equation:

$$E = mc^2$$

In the equation, if E is energy in joules, then c (the speed of light) must be 3×10^8 m/s, and m (the mass) must be measured in kilograms.

EXERCISES

1. Which of the following equations can be used to compute the mass equivalence of an x-ray photon?
   a. $m = Ec^2$
   b. $m = zv^2$
   c. $m = E/c^2$
   d. $m = \frac{1}{2} E^2$
   e. $m = Ev$

2. Which of the following equations can be used to compute the mass equivalence of an x-ray if its frequency is known?
   a. $m = E/c^2$
   b. $m = Ec^2$
   c. $m = hf/c^2$
   d. $m = h/\lambda f$
   e. $m = \frac{1}{2} c^2$

3. In the case of mass-energy conversions:
   a. Nuclear fission is an example.
   b. The inverse square law applies.
   c. The law of conservation of energy is violated.
   d. The law of conservation of matter is violated.
   e. The wave equation is an example.

4. In Einstein's relativistic equation, $E = mc^2$:
   a. c represents the velocity of ultrasound.
   b. If the mass is measured in kilograms and the velocity in meters per second, energy will be measured in joules.
   c. If the mass is measured in grams, the velocity must be measured in meters per second.
   d. If the velocity is 3×10^8 m/s, mass should be in grams.
   e. If the velocity is given as 186,000 miles/s, the energy will be in newtons.

5. When Einstein's relativistic equation is used to compute the energy equivalence of matter, it is usual to express such energy in:
   a. Calories
   b. Coulombs
   c. Ergs
   d. Joules
   e. Newtons

6. Energy can be:
   a. Created but not destroyed
   b. Destroyed but not created
   c. Expressed in newtons
   d. Measured in grays
   e. Transformed into matter

7. The energy equivalence of an electron at rest is 511 keV. It is also:
   a. 511 eV
   b. 511 MeV
   c. 0.51 eV
   d. 0.51 MeV
   e. 5.1 MeV

8. When various types of radiation are compared:
   a. The mass equivalence of a television broadcast is greater than that of red light.
   b. The mass equivalence of an FM broadcast is greater than that of ultraviolet light.
   c. The mass equivalence of blue light is greater than that of red light.
   d. The mass equivalence of microwaves is greater than that of x-rays.
   e. The mass equivalence of red light is greater than that of ultraviolet light.

9. If the entire mass of an electron ($m = 9.1 \times 10^{-31}$ kg) could be converted into an x-ray, its energy would be approximately:
   a. 4.15×10^{-15} eV-s
   b. 4.15×10^{-15} keV-s
   c. 511,000 eV
   d. 511 eV
   e. 5.1 MeV

10. One amu equals 1.66×10^{-27} kg. Its energy equivalence is:
    a. 1.5×10^{-10} J
    b. 1.5×10^{-7} J
    c. 1.5 kJ
    d. 1.5 mJ
    e. 1.5 nJ

11. What is the mass equivalence of a 35 keV x-ray?
    a. 6.3×10^{-31} kg
    b. 6.3×10^{-32} kg
    c. 6.3×10^{-33} kg
    d. 6.3×10^{-34} kg
    e. 6.3×10^{-35} kg

12. The SI unit for energy is the:
    a. Dyne
    b. Electron volt
    c. Erg
    d. Joule
    e. Newton

13. The energy of a 70 keV x-ray can be expressed as:
    a. 1.1×10^{-16} J
    b. 1.1×10^{-14} J
    c. 1.1×10^{-12} J
    d. 1.1×10^{-10} J
    e. 1.1×10^{-9} J

14. The equivalence of mass and energy is described by:
    a. The Bohr constant
    b. Einstein's theory
    c. Joule's laws
    d. Newton's laws
    e. Planck's theory

15. The energy of diagnostic x-rays is similar to that of which of the following radiations?
    a. Diffraction x-rays
    b. Grenz x-rays
    c. Megavoltage radiation
    d. Orthovoltage x-rays
    e. Superficial x-rays

16. In the equation $E = hf$, the h:
    a. Has units of energy
    b. Is a variable
    c. Stands for the Einstein constant
    d. Stands for the Bohr constant
    e. Relates photon energy to frequency

17. Planck's constant (h) has units of:
    a. eVs
    b. eVm/s
    c. JeV
    d. Jm
    e. Jm/s

18. Longer-wavelength x-rays have:
    a. Higher energy
    b. Higher mass
    c. Higher velocity
    d. Lower energy
    e. Lower velocity

Worksheet 5-1 Electrostatics

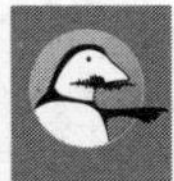

Matter has mass and energy equivalence. Matter may also have an electric charge.

Electrostatics is the study of stationary electric charges:

- Electrified objects have excess charges.
- Objects can be electrified by contact, friction, or induction.
- Opposite charges attract; like charges repel.
- The magnitude of the attraction or repulsion is given by Coulomb's law:

$$F = k\frac{Q_a Q_b}{d^2}$$

where F is the force in newtons (attractive or repulsive), Q_a and Q_b are electrostatic charges in coulombs, d is separation distance in meters, and k is the proportionality constant ($k = 9.0 \times 10^9 N - m^2/C^2$).

EXERCISES

1. What is the principal reservoir for the excess electric charge?
   a. Clouds
   b. Lightning rod
   c. The atmosphere
   d. The Earth
   e. Water pipes

2. Regarding the movement of an electric charge from one atom to another atom:
   a. Both positive and negative charges can move.
   b. It must occur in a large atom.
   c. Only positive charges move.
   d. Usually inner-shell electrons move.
   e. Usually outer-shell electrons move.

3. Electric energy can be converted into:
   a. Chemical energy by an x-ray imaging system
   b. Electromagnetic energy by a battery
   c. Mechanical energy by a battery
   d. Nuclear energy in a nuclear reactor
   e. Thermal energy by a lamp

4. Electrostatics:
   a. Concerns resting electric charges
   b. Concerns the mass-energy conversion of electrons
   c. Governs the movement of electric charges in a conductor
   d. Is the conversion of kinetic energy
   e. Is the study of photon radiation

5. Coulomb's law states that electrostatic force is:
   a. Dependent on mAs
   b. Directly proportional to the square of the distance between charges
   c. Directly proportional to the square of the product of charges
   d. Inversely proportional to the product of charges
   e. Inversely proportional to the square of the distance between charges

6. Which of the following is a method of electrification?
   a. Diffraction
   b. Excitation
   c. Induction
   d. Resonance
   e. Transmission

7. Static electricity:
   a. Can make one's hair stand on end
   b. Can produce x-rays
   c. Can result in magnetism
   d. Is the basis for transformer operation
   e. Is the study of electric currents

8. The unit of electrostatic charge is the:
   a. Ampere
   b. Coulomb
   c. Electron volt
   d. Newton
   e. Volt

9. The principal electrostatic law states that:
   a. A neutron will repel a neutron.
   b. A proton will repel a neutron.
   c. An electron will repel a neutron.
   d. An electron will repel a proton.
   e. An electron will repel an electron.

10. Objects become electrified because of:
    a. An excess of neutrons
    b. An excess of protons
    c. The transfer of electrons
    d. The transfer of neutrons
    e. The transfer of protons

11. The phenomenon of lightning occurs when:
    a. Adjacent clouds are electrically neutral.
    b. Adjacent clouds have negative electrification.
    c. Adjacent clouds have positive electrification.
    d. One cloud is positively electrified and an adjacent one is negatively electrified.
    e. Thunder is heard.

12. Which of the following would be included as one of the four basic electrostatic laws?
    a. Archimedes' principle
    b. Conversion to magnetism
    c. Einstein's law
    d. Electric charge concentration
    e. Planck's law

13. An electrostatic force is created when a/an:
    a. Electrostatic charge exists.
    b. Neutron approaches a neutron.
    c. Neutron approaches an electron.
    d. Proton approaches a neutron.
    e. Proton approaches a proton.

14. A radiographic tube is operated at 500 mA. How many electrons per second is this?
    a. 3.2×10^{9}
    b. 3.2×10^{18}
    c. 6.3×10^{9}
    d. 6.3×10^{17}
    e. 6.3×10^{18}

15. The unit of electrostatic force is the:
    a. Coulomb
    b. Electron volt
    c. Joule
    d. Newton
    e. Gray

16. Which of the following are *not* affected by electrostatically charged matter?
    a. Alpha particles
    b. Beta particles
    c. Electrons
    d. Protons
    e. X-rays

17. How many electrons are contained in 0.5 μC?
    a. 3.2×10^{6}
    b. 3.2×10^{12}
    c. 6.3×10^{6}
    d. 6.3×10^{12}
    e. 6.3×10^{18}

18. When a copper conductor becomes electrified:
    a. A kink in the wire will have the lowest surface electrification.
    b. Excess electrons are uniformly distributed throughout the wire.
    c. It becomes heated.
    d. Negative charges concentrate on the surface, and positive charges are distributed throughout.
    e. The distribution of protons on its surface is uniform.

19. The unit of electric potential is the:
    a. Ampere
    b. Coulomb
    c. Newton
    d. Ohm
    e. Volt

20. Two positive 0.5 C charges are positioned 1.0 m apart. The force acting between them is:
    a. Attractive
    b. Exponential
    c. Neutral
    d. Repulsive
    e. Variable

Worksheet 5-2 Electrodynamics

Electrodynamics is the study of electric charge in motion. A conductor is any material through which electrons flow easily. An insulator is any material that does not allow electron flow. A semiconductor is a material that under some conditions behaves as an insulator and under other conditions behaves as a conductor. A superconductor conducts electrons with no electrical resistance.

OHM'S LAW

Ohm's law: $V = IR$, where V is the electric potential in volts, I is the electric current in amperes, and R is the electric resistance in ohms (Ω).

Series circuits

Total resistance: $R_T = R_1 + R_2 + R_3 \ldots$

Total current: $I_T = I_1 + I_2 + I_3 \ldots$

Total voltage: $V_T = V_1 + V_2 + V_3 \ldots$

Parallel circuits

Total resistance: $\frac{1}{R_T} = \frac{1}{R_1} + \frac{1}{R_2} + \frac{1}{R} + \ldots$

Total current: $I_T = I_1 + I_2 + I_3 + \ldots$

Total voltage: $V_T = V_1 = V_2 = V_3 \ldots$

EXERCISES

1. Which of the following is the best electric insulator?
   a. Aluminum
   b. Copper
   c. Nickel
   d. Water
   e. Wood

2. The ratio of the electric potential across a circuit element to the current flowing through that element is called:
   a. Current
   b. Energy
   c. Power
   d. Resistance
   e. Voltage

3. The electrical resistance of the wire increases as the diameter of the:
   a. Insulator decreases
   b. Insulator increases
   c. Power supply increases
   d. Wire decreases
   e. Wire increases

4. When an electric current flows through a wire with resistance (R), energy is:
   a. Absorbed as heat
   b. Absorbed as light
   c. Generated as heat
   d. Generated as x-rays
   e. Transformed to mass

5. When electrons move in a copper wire:
   a. Resistance to the electron flow exists.
   b. Ionization occurs.
   c. The condition is called electromagnetic force.
   d. The condition is called electrostatics.
   e. They move down the middle of the wire.

6. The number of volts required to cause a current of 40 A in a circuit having a resistance of 5 Ω is:
   a. 5 V
   b. 8 V
   c. 40 V
   d. 45 V
   e. 200 V

7. The unit of electric potential is the:
   a. Ampere
   b. Coulomb
   c. Joule
   d. Ohm
   e. Volt

8. Ohm's law states that:
   a. Electric current is the product of voltage and resistance.
   b. Electric power is equal to current squared times voltage.
   c. Electric power is equal to voltage times current.
   d. The electric potential is equal to the current squared times resistance.
   e. The electric potential is the product of current and resistance.

9. The flow of 1 C/s in a conductor is equal to:
   a. 1 Ω
   b. 1 A
   c. 1 eV
   d. 1 kVp
   e. 1 V

10. In a series circuit:
    a. Ohm's law fails.
    b. Only three circuit elements are allowed.
    c. The total current is the sum of the individual currents.
    d. The total resistance is the sum of the individual resistances.
    e. The voltage drop across each circuit element is the same.

11. In electrodynamics, which of the following is a *correct* expression?
    a. $I = Qt$
    b. $R = I^2V$
    c. $R = IV$
    d. $V = IR$
    e. $V = I/R$

12. Which of the following is normally measured in volts?
    a. Electric potential
    b. Electromagnetic force
    c. Electromagnetic potential
    d. Electromagnetic radiation
    e. Electrostatic force

13. Milliampere-seconds (mAs) is a unit of:
    a. Electric current
    b. Electric potential
    c. Electromagnetic force
    d. Electromotive force
    e. Electrostatic charge

14. Electric insulators:
    a. Consist of materials such as silicon and germanium
    b. Convert electric energy to electromagnetic energy
    c. Convert electric energy to heat
    d. Inhibit movement of electric charge
    e. Permit movement of electric charge

15. 1 A is equal to:
    a. 1 Ω/s
    b. 1 C/s
    c. 1 eV/s
    d. 1 J/s
    e. 1 V/s

Worksheet 5-3 Alternating and Direct Currents

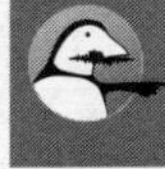

- Direct current (DC), which is usually provided by a battery, flows in one direction.
- Alternating current (AC) supplies power at 60 Hz.
- Electric power is measured in watts (W).

$$P = VI$$

$$\text{Power (W)} = \text{Voltage (V)} \times \text{Current (I)}$$

and

$$P = I^2R$$

$$\text{Power (W) (Current [I]}^2 \times \text{ Resistance [R])}$$

and

$$E = Pt$$

$$\text{Electric energy (J)} = \text{Power (W)} \times \text{Time (S)}$$

EXERCISES

1. The distinct difference between AC and DC is that:
   a. DC can attain higher current.
   b. DC can attain higher voltage.
   c. DC electron flow is in one direction.
   d. DC electron flow varies in amplitude.
   e. DC has higher electrical resistance.

2. If a 60 W lightbulb is operated at 120 V, the current flowing through the bulb is approximately:
   a. 0.5 A
   b. 1 A
   c. 50 A
   d. 100 A
   e. 500 A

3. An x-ray imaging system has a 30 kW generator. If the maximum tube voltage is 150 kV, what is the available tube current?
   a. 200 mA
   b. 400 mA
   c. 600 mA
   d. 2 A
   e. 5 A

4. If a sine curve is used to represent 60 Hz AC, then:
   a. During the negative half-cycle, there is no electron flow.
   b. The amplitude of the curve is directly related to wavelength.
   c. The time from a positive peak to the next negative valley is 8 ms.
   d. The time from zero crossing to maximum amplitude is one cycle.
   e. The time from zero crossing to maximum amplitude is one-half cycle.

5. When electricity exists as 60 Hz AC:
   a. Electrons flow in one direction in alternating bursts.
   b. Electrons flow randomly in both directions.
   c. The number of electrons is proportional to the voltage.
   d. The velocity of electron flow is proportional to the current.
   e. The velocity of electron flow is proportional to the voltage.

6. In the United States, normal household electric power is:
   a. 50 V, 120 Hz, three-phase
   b. 60 V, 120 Hz, single-phase
   c. 120 V, 50 Hz, three-phase
   d. 120 V, 60 Hz, single-phase
   e. 120 V, 60 Hz, three-phase

7. The unit of electric power is the:
   a. Hertz
   b. Joule
   c. Newton
   d. Volt
   e. Watt

8. Electricity is purchased on the basis of the kilowatt-hours one consumes. The kilowatt-hour also can be expressed in the unit:
   a. Amperes per second
   b. Joule
   c. Newton
   d. Volt
   e. Watts per ampere

9. Which of the following equations can be used to calculate electric power (P) consumption?
   a. $P = I^2V$
   b. $P = IR$
   c. $P = IV$
   d. $P = VR$
   e. $P = V/R$

10. A hair dryer is rated at 1000 W. Approximately what current will it produce on a normal 120 V, 60 Hz AC household supply?
   a. 8 A
   b. 10 A
   c. 80 A
   d. 110 A
   e. 800 A

Worksheet 5-4 Magnetism

- There are three states of magnetism: ferromagnetic, paramagnetic, and diamagnetic. Strongly magnetized material is ferromagnetic. Weakly magnetized material is paramagnetic. Nonmagnetic material is diamagnetic.
- The degree of magnetism increases as the number of unpaired electrons in an atom increases.
- Magnetic permeability is the property of a material to attract magnetic field lines.
- Magnetic susceptibility is the ease with which a material can be rendered magnetic.

EXERCISES

1. Which of the following is a physical property that we cannot sense?
   a. Acceleration
   b. Electric current
   c. Heat
   d. Magnetism
   e. Mass

2. An example of a magnetic domain is:
   a. A bar magnet
   b. A nucleus
   c. A permanent magnet
   d. An electromagnet
   e. The Earth

3. If a bar magnet were suspended in space and another bar of nonmagnetic material were brought close to it, what would happen?
   a. Nothing.
   b. The bar magnet would be attracted.
   c. The bar magnet would become demagnetized.
   d. The bar magnet would rotate.
   e. The imaginary magnetic field lines would be deviated.

4. If two bar magnets suspended in space were brought together, what would happen?
   a. Nothing.
   b. One would rotate.
   c. The north pole of one would point to the north pole of the other.
   d. They would rotate and attract.
   e. They would rotate and repel.

5. A lodestone is an example of:
   a. A magnetic domain
   b. A natural magnet
   c. An electromagnet
   d. Demagnetized matter
   e. Paramagnetism

6. Which of the following would likely be classified as ferromagnetic material?
   a. Air
   b. Glass
   c. Iron
   d. Lead
   e. Water

7. If two magnets are brought together, north-to-north poles will ________, whereas north-to-south poles will ________.
   a. Attract; attract
   b. Attract; repel
   c. Not interact; interact
   d. Repel; attract
   e. Repel; repel

8. Most magnets:
   a. Are affected by another magnetic field
   b. Are diamagnetic
   c. Are naturally occurring if used in science and technology
   d. Have north, south, and neutral poles
   e. Have positive, negative, and neutral poles

9. Most magnetic materials are:
   a. Also radioactive
   b. Attracted to copper
   c. Bar shaped
   d. Shaped like a horseshoe
   e. Still magnetic when broken

10. A navigational compass:
    a. Has a north pole that is attracted to the equator
    b. Has a north pole that is attracted to the magnetic north pole of the Earth
    c. Has both a north and a south pole
    d. Is usually made of glass
    e. Will not work at the equator

11. Which of the following is a classification of magnetism?
    a. Coulombic
    b. Diploic
    c. Electromagnetism
    d. Paramagnetism
    e. Polar magnetism

12. The Earth's magnetic field is strongest:
    a. At the equator
    b. At the poles
    c. In deep space
    d. In near space
    e. In the atmosphere above the equator

13. The physical laws of magnetism:
    a. Include the conversion to electricity.
    b. Include the conservation of magnetism.
    c. Require that there be a south pole for every north pole.
    d. Require that there be a south pole for every north pole but only for magnets of certain shapes.
    e. Specify a force that increases with increasing distance from the magnet

14. Which of the following can create a magnetic field?
    a. A neutron at rest
    b. A quantum of visible light
    c. A spinning proton
    d. A stable atom
    e. An x-ray

15. The force between the poles of two bar magnets:
    a. Depends on the permeability of matter separating the magnets.
    b. Is inversely proportional to the strength of each magnet.
    c. Obeys a law similar in form to Planck's law.
    d. Obeys the inverse square law.
    e. Varies directly with the distance between them.

16. When iron is fabricated into a magnet, magnetic domains:
    a. Align
    b. Cancel
    c. Disappear
    d. Induce
    e. Magnify

17. Magnetism has some properties similar to those of electrostatics, such as:
    a. Both can be converted to mass.
    b. Both can be sensed by touch.
    c. Both involve proton-type radiation.
    d. Both obey the inverse square law.
    e. Both refer to iron substances.

18. Magnetism:
    a. Can be converted to electricity.
    b. Depends on monopolar atoms.
    c. Is defined as a property that can attract glass, wood, or metal.
    d. Is present in some naturally occurring ores.
    e. Requires electricity.

19. When a charged particle moves in a straight line, a magnetic field is:
    a. Created along the direction of particle motion.
    b. Created and has the same sign as the particle.
    c. Created perpendicular to the particle motion.
    d. Erased.
    e. Reversed.

20. Which of the following has an associated magnetic field?
    a. Helium atom
    b. A Styrofoam cup
    c. Hydrogen nucleus
    d. Neutron
    e. Stationary electron

21. When iron is brought near a permanent magnet, the lines of the magnetic field are:
    a. Attracted to the iron
    b. Attracted to the magnet
    c. Repelled by the iron
    d. Repelled by the magnet
    e. Unaffected

Worksheet 5-5 Electromagnetic Effect Electromagnetic Induction

A current-carrying coil of wire creates a magnetic field. If an iron core is inserted, the magnetic field becomes many times more intense because the magnetic permeability of iron is greater than that of air. Such a device is called an *electromagnet*. Electromagnets are used in some x-ray imaging systems as switches.

EXERCISES

1. An electron moving in a conductor:
   a. Causes the conductor to behave as a bar magnet
   b. Causes the conductor to bend
   c. Produces a magnetic field in the conductor
   d. Produces a magnetic field perpendicular to the conductor
   e. Produces light in the conductor

2. The voltaic pile:
   a. Consists of a magnet and a conductor
   b. Consists of a pile of charges
   c. Consists of zinc and copper plates sandwiched together
   d. Is a modern dry-cell battery
   e. Was invented by Faraday

3. Electromotive force (EMF):
   a. Is an electrical mechanical force
   b. Is expressed in joules
   c. Is expressed in volts
   d. Stands for electromagnetic field
   e. Was discovered by Hans Oersted

4. The experimental link connecting electric and magnetic forces was discovered by:
   a. Edison
   b. Faraday
   c. Lenz
   d. Oersted
   e. Volta

5. The device designed to measure electron flow in a conductor is known as a/an:
   a. Ammeter
   b. Choke coil
   c. Electromagnet
   d. Solenoid
   e. Voltmeter

6. The fact that an electric current is induced if the conductor is in a changing magnetic field:
   a. Is known as Faraday's law
   b. Is known as Ohm's law
   c. Is the statement of the second law of electromagnetics
   d. Was discovered by Lenz
   e. Was discovered by Volta

7. The term *electromagnetic induction* refers to the production of:
   a. A magnetic field
   b. A static charge
   c. An electric current
   d. An electromagnet
   e. Electromagnetic radiation

8. A difference between self-induction and mutual induction is that:
   a. Mutual induction is the basis for an electric motor and self-induction is the basis for a transformer.
   b. Mutual induction requires two coils and self-induction requires only one.
   c. Only self-induction can create EMF.
   d. Self-induction requires two coils and mutual induction requires only one.
   e. There is no difference.

9. The magnetic field produced by an electromagnet has:
   a. Alternating poles
   b. Neither a North nor a South pole
   c. Only a North pole
   d. Only a South pole
   e. Properties similar to a bar magnet

10. One law of electromagnetics states that:
    a. An electric current is induced in a circuit if some part of that circuit is in a magnetic field.
    b. Electrostatics can be converted to magnetism.
    c. The induced current flows in the opposite direction of the inducing action.
    d. The right-hand rule is used to determine the direction of the induced current.
    e. There are two basic types of induction: primary and secondary.

11. The magnetic field produced:
    a. By a solenoid is more intense than that produced by an electromagnet
    b. By AC is stronger than that produced by DC
    c. By an AC source is constant
    d. In a transformer is based on mutual induction
    e. In an electromagnet is most intense in the plane perpendicular to its axis
12. An electromagnet:
    a. Cannot be turned off
    b. Has an air core
    c. Is a coil of wire wound around an iron core
    d. Produces a magnetic field with or without an electric current
    e. Produces a monopolar magnetic field
13. Given a closed loop of wire with no electron flow, an electric current can be induced if:
    a. A changing magnetic field is present.
    b. A constant magnetic field is present.
    c. No magnetic field is present.
    d. The loop is cycled open/closed.
    e. The loop is opened.
14. When an AC source is connected to a coil of wire:
    a. A constant magnetic field is generated.
    b. A front EMF is produced.
    c. An opposite EMF is induced.
    d. Electromagnetic radiation is produced.
    e. Mutual induction occurs.
15. When an electric current is induced by mutual induction, such current flows:
    a. According to Faraday's law
    b. According to Lenz's law
    c. According to Oersted's law
    d. In the primary coil
    e. In the secondary coil
16. Which of the following scientists is associated with the early development of electromagnetism?
    a. Edison
    b. Faraday
    c. Marconi
    d. Planck
    e. Roentgen
17. A modern dry-cell battery is a source of:
    a. Coulomb per joule
    b. Joule per coulomb
    c. Newton per coulomb
    d. Ohm per volt
    e. Volt per ohm
18. When the right-hand rule is applied to a straight wire, the thumb indicates the direction of the:
    a. Circuit resistance
    b. Electric current
    c. Electric field
    d. Electric potential
    e. Magnetic field
19. The principal difference between a solenoid and an electromagnet in a magnetic field:
    a. Homogeneity
    b. Intensity
    c. Penetrability
    d. Polarity
    e. Variability
20. Which of the following is based on electromagnetic induction?
    a. AC current
    b. Battery
    c. DC current
    d. Radio reception
    e. Solenoid

Worksheet 5-6 Electromagnetic Devices

A coil of wire is called a solenoid. When the coil of wire is wrapped around an iron core, the generated magnetic field is intensified. Such a device is an electromagnet.

Electric generators and motors are electromechanical devices. The former converts mechanical energy to electric energy; the latter converts electric energy to mechanical energy.

Electric motors operate by passing an electric current through a loop of wire while in the presence of a magnetic field. The interaction between the electric current and the fixed magnetic field causes the loop to rotate, thereby producing mechanical energy. The induction motor, which is a type of electric motor, is used in all rotating anode x-ray tubes.

EXERCISES

1. Which of the following is *most* related to electromechanical devices?
   a. Edison's law of electromechanics
   b. Faraday's experiment
   c. Lenz's first law of electromagnetics
   d. Oersted's experiment on mutual induction
   e. The voltaic pile

2. In an electric generator:
   a. A coil of wire is rotated in a magnetic field.
   b. A transformer is charged.
   c. Alternating current (AC) is changed to direct current (DC).
   d. Chemical energy is converted to electrical energy.
   e. Electrical energy is converted to mechanical energy.

3. The electric generator is *most* closely associated with experiments conducted by:
   a. Edison
   b. Faraday
   c. Lenz
   d. Oersted
   e. Volta

4. Which of the following statements about generators and motors is always *true?*
   a. They are electromagnets.
   b. They both require commutators.
   c. They convert energy from one form into another.
   d. They have both primary and secondary windings.
   e. They require direct electric contact between primary and secondary coils.

5. In an electric motor:
   a. A coil of wire is mechanically rotated.
   b. A commutator ring is not necessary.
   c. AC is changed to DC.
   d. A transformer is discharged.
   e. Electric current is supplied to a coil of wire.

6. Which of the following would be classified as electromechanical devices?
   a. Generators and motors
   b. Generators and rectifiers
   c. Motors and rectifiers
   d. Transformers and electromagnets
   e. Transformers and rectifiers

7. The main difference between an AC and a DC electric generator is:
   a. The type of commutator ring
   b. A magnet
   c. A source of electromotive force
   d. A transformer
   e. A voltmeter

8. The electric current produced by an AC generator has:
   a. Alternating positive and negative intensity
   b. Constant negative intensity
   c. Constant positive intensity
   d. Pulsating negative intensity
   e. Pulsating positive intensity

9. An induction motor is used in an x-ray imaging system to:
   a. Control current
   b. Measure mAs
   c. Provide rectification
   d. Rotate the anode
   e. Vary voltage

10. In an induction motor, the only part to be rotated is the:
    a. Cathode
    b. Electromagnet
    c. Rotor
    d. Stator
    e. Wire loop

11. A fluoroscope is operated at 95 kVp, 2 mA. What is its power consumption?
    a. 47.5 W
    b. 190 W
    c. 47.5 kW
    d. 97 kW
    e. 190 kW

12. What power is required for radiographic exposure at 76 kVp, 500 mA?
    a. 19 W
    b. 380 W
    c. 576 W
    d. 19 kW
    e. 38 kW

13. A 110 V heater requires 15 A. What is the power consumption?
    a. 15 W
    b. 110 W
    c. 125 W
    d. 1650 W
    e. 1800 W

14. How much current will a 60 W lightbulb draw from a 120 V receptacle?
    a. 60 mA
    b. 500 mA
    c. 1 A
    d. 15 A
    e. 120 A

15. Electric current waveforms are graphs of:
    a. Electric current versus resistance
    b. Electric current versus time
    c. Electric current versus voltage
    d. Electric voltage versus current
    e. Electric voltage versus resistance

16. Theoretically, conduction electrons come to rest momentarily:
    a. At the peak of the waveform
    b. At the valley of the waveform
    c. At zero crossing
    d. Just before either a peak or a valley
    e. They never come to rest

17. Electric ranges, air conditioners, and furnaces require 220 V, 60 Hz AC. Therefore compared with most household appliances, they require which of the following?
    a. A higher electric potential
    b. A higher operating frequency
    c. A lower electric potential
    d. Greater conductivity
    e. Greater semiconductivity

Worksheet 5-7
The Transformer

A transformer consists of two electromagnets with a common iron core. A voltage impressed on the primary coil will generate a voltage in the secondary coil, provided that the power is AC. The transformer law is as follows:

$$\frac{V_s}{V_p} = \frac{N_s}{N_p}$$

where the subscript s refers to the secondary coil, the subscript p refers to the primary coil, N is the number of turns of the coil, and V is the voltage. The ratio N_s/N_p is known as the **turns ratio**.

In an x-ray imaging system, there are usually three transformers: the variable-voltage autotransformer, the high-voltage step-up transformer, and the step-down filament transformer.

EXERCISES

1. The transformer changes:
   a. Electric current to voltage
   b. Electric energy to electromagnetic energy
   c. Electric energy to mechanical energy
   d. Mechanical energy to electric energy
   e. The amplitude of the voltage

2. A transformer operates:
   a. On AC but not on DC
   b. On both DC and AC
   c. On DC but not on AC
   d. Only above its critical current
   e. Only on a constant voltage

3. If a transformer produces a large secondary current from a small primary current:
   a. Power will be increased.
   b. The turns ratio will be greater than 1.
   c. The turns ratio will be less than 1.
   d. The voltage will be larger on the secondary side than on the primary side.
   e. There will be more windings on the secondary side than on the primary side.

4. The principal application of a transformer in an x-ray imaging system is to:
   a. Change AC to DC
   b. Change DC to AC
   c. Change frequency
   d. Change voltage
   e. Produce x-rays

5. The output current in a step-up transformer is:
   a. Higher than the input current
   b. Independent of the input current
   c. Independent of the turns ratio
   d. Lower than the input current
   e. The same as the input current

6. A transformer with a turns ratio of 1000:1 is:
   a. A step-down transformer
   b. A step-up transformer
   c. An autotransformer
   d. Used to increase current
   e. Used to reduce voltage

7. When a step-up transformer is in use:
   a. The primary winding has more turns than the secondary winding.
   b. The secondary current is greater than the primary current.
   c. The secondary voltage is greater than the primary voltage.
   d. X-ray tube current is selected.
   e. The turns ratio is equal to 1.

8. When a transformer is designed, the change in current is:
   a. Dependent on the supply voltage
   b. Directly proportional to the voltage change
   c. In the same direction as the voltage change
   d. Inversely proportional to the turns ratio
   e. Proportional to the turns ratio

9. Which of the following is a transformer design used in x-ray imaging systems?
   a. Capacitor type
   b. Filament type
   c. Rectifier type
   d. Rotating type
   e. Shell type

10. An autotransformer:
    a. Contains a single coil that serves as both primary and secondary coils
    b. Controls x-ray tube current
    c. Is a shell type of transformer
    d. Is an electromechanical device
    e. Is used to control the frequency

11. Which of the following statements about transformers is *correct?*
    a. If there were equal numbers of primary and secondary coil turns, the turns ratio would be zero.
    b. In the shell-type transformer, the primary and secondary coils are wound on different cores.
    c. Laminated transformer cores are more efficient than unlaminated ones.
    d. The autotransformer controls current.
    e. The high-voltage transformer in an x-ray imaging system is the autotransformer.

12. A transformer "transforms" or changes electric:
    a. Frequency
    b. Impedance
    c. Power
    d. Resistance
    e. Voltage

13. Transformers have iron cores to intensify the:
    a. Electric current
    b. Electric potential
    c. Electric power
    d. Electric voltage
    e. Magnetic field

14. Primary to secondary coupling in a transformer is enhanced by:
    a. 60 Hz
    b. AC
    c. An iron core
    d. DC
    e. EMF

15. If DC is applied to the primary coil of a step-up transformer, what is the result in the secondary coil?
    a. AC
    b. Increased current
    c. Increased magnetic field
    d. Increased voltage
    e. Nothing

16. The *turns ratio* is defined as:
    a. Number of secondary windings ÷ primary windings
    b. Primary iron core ÷ secondary iron core
    c. Primary voltage ÷ secondary voltage
    d. Primary windings ÷ number of secondary windings
    e. Secondary current ÷ primary current

17. Which of the following accurately represents the transformer law?
    a. $I_s/I_p = N_p/N_s$
    b. $I_s/I_p = N_s/N_p$
    c. $I_s/I_p = V_s/V_p$
    d. $I_p/I_s = V_p/V_s$
    e. $I_p/I_s = N_p/N_s$

18. What is the transformer that looks like a square doughnut called?
    a. Auto
    b. Closed core
    c. High frequency
    d. Induction
    e. Shell type

Worksheet 6-1 Operating Console Control of Kilovolt Peak (kVp)

- Peak kilovoltage (kVp) is controlled by a series of electric taps on the autotransformer.
- The autotransformer has only one winding.
- The autotransformer can function in the step-up or the step-down mode.
- The transformer law can be used to calculate the secondary voltage:

$$\frac{V_s}{V_p} = \frac{N_s}{N_p}$$

where V_p refers to primary voltage, V_s is secondary voltage, N_p refers to the number of windings enclosed by primary taps, and N_s is the number of windings enclosed by secondary taps.

EXERCISES

1. Power to the primary side of the high-voltage transformer comes from the:
   a. Filament transformer
   b. Line-voltage compensator
   c. Primary side of the autotransformer
   d. Rectifier
   e. Secondary side of the autotransformer

2. The output voltage from the autotransformer is:
   a. Always less than the input voltage
   b. Always more than the input voltage
   c. Fed directly to the rectifiers
   d. Inversely proportional to the turns ratio
   e. Proportional to the turns ratio

3. The autotransformer converts:
   a. Chemical energy to electric energy
   b. Electric energy to chemical energy
   c. Electric energy to electric energy
   d. Magnetic energy to electric energy
   e. Mechanical energy to electric energy

4. The autotransformer operates on the principle of:
   a. Coulomb's law
   b. Edison's law
   c. Faraday's law
   d. Newton's law
   e. Oersted's law

5. The principal purpose of the high-voltage transformer is to do which of the following?
   a. Adjust voltage
   b. Increase voltage
   c. Rectify voltage
   d. Reduce voltage
   e. Stabilize voltage

6. The voltage supplied to an x-ray imaging system is 220 V. The voltage used by the x-ray tube is produced by which of the following?
   a. Autotransformer
   b. Exposure timer
   c. Filament transformer
   d. High-voltage transformer
   e. Rheostat

7. 220 V is supplied to 800 primary turns of an autotransformer. What will be the output voltage across 200 secondary turns?
   a. 27.5 V
   b. 50 V
   c. 880 V
   d. 1760 V
   e. 3520 V

8. The autotransformer has only one:
   a. Coil
   b. Meter
   c. Rectifier
   d. Switch
   e. Turns ratio

9. The principal purpose of the autotransformer is to:
   a. Adjust voltage
   b. Increase voltage
   c. Rectify voltage
   d. Reduce voltage
   e. Stabilize voltage

10. Which of the following is directly connected to the autotransformer?
    a. Filament
    b. kVp meter
    c. mA meter
    d. Rectifier
    e. X-ray tube

11. Taps on the windings of an autotransformer are used to select which of the following?
    a. Exposure time
    b. Focal spot
    c. Line compensation
    d. mA
    e. Rectification

12. 440 V is supplied to 1000 primary turns of an autotransformer. If the desired output voltage is 100 V, how many secondary turns must be tapped?
    a. 100
    b. 250
    c. 454
    d. 4400
    e. 10,000

13. The autotransformer can be used to do which of the following?
    a. Control exposure time
    b. Convert AC to DC
    c. Convert DC to AC
    d. Increase kVp
    e. Increase mA

14. If V stands for voltage and T for the number of turns enclosed between the taps of an autotransformer, then the autotransformer law is which of the following?
    a. $V_p/V_s = T_p/T_s$
    b. $V_p T_p = T_s V_s$
    c. $V_p V_s = T_p T_s$
    d. $V_s/V_p = T_p/T_s$
    e. $V_s = V_p$

15. In the design of an autotransformer:
    a. A single coil serves as both the primary and the secondary coils.
    b. The exposure timer is on the primary side.
    c. The major kVp adjustment and the line-voltage compensator are on the secondary side.
    d. The major kVp adjustment is on the primary side, and the minor kVp adjustment is on the secondary side.
    e. There are separate primary and secondary coils.

16. Selection of kVp:
    a. Involves two series of autotransformers
    b. Requires rectified voltage
    c. Requires that constant voltage be supplied to the autotransformer
    d. Uses meters and switches that are at high kVp
    e. Uses the step-up transformer

17. Line compensation:
    a. Adjusts the line frequency to 60 Hz
    b. Compensates for rectification
    c. Is necessary for proper exposure timing
    d. Is necessary to convert AC to DC
    e. Is required to stabilize voltage

18. Which of the following is used to determine the voltage before exposure?
    a. A filament transformer
    b. A postreading voltmeter
    c. A prereading voltmeter
    d. A step-up transformer
    e. An autotransformer

Worksheet 6-2 Operating Console Control of Milliamperage (mA)

The x-ray tube current is controlled by an electric filament circuit that is separated from the high-voltage circuit. The important circuit elements for supplying and controlling the tube mA are the autotransformer, the precision resistors, the filament transformer, and the filament.

The mA meter, although physically located on the operating console, is electrically connected to the secondary side of the high-voltage transformer through a center tap to the electrical ground. This allows for direct measurement of the tube current without the possibility of electric shock.

Thermionic emission is the release of electrons from a heated filament. A correction circuit is incorporated to control the **space charge effect**.

EXERCISES

1. One coulomb per second (C/s) is equivalent to 1 A, and 1 C is equal to 6.3×10^{18} electrons. Therefore operation at 100 mA would result in a current of:
   a. 6.3×10^{16} electrons
   b. 6.3×10^{16} electrons/s
   c. 6.3×10^{17} electrons
   d. 6.3×10^{17} electrons/s
   e. 6.3×10^{18} electrons

2. The filament transformer:
   a. Has four windings
   b. Increases current
   c. Increases voltage
   d. Is an autotransformer
   e. Must have precision resistors

3. The filament transformer is usually:
   a. A part of the autotransformer
   b. Located with the high-voltage generator
   c. An autotransformer
   d. Located in the operating console
   e. A step-down transformer

4. A posteroanterior chest requires a technique of 125 kVp at 4 mAs. The total number of electrons used to make the exposure is:
   a. 2.5×10^{15}
   b. 2.5×10^{16}
   c. 2.5×10^{17}
   d. 6.3×10^{16}
   e. 6.3×10^{17}

5. The filament circuit:
   a. Begins at the filament and ends at the filament transformer
   b. Begins at the autotransformer and ends at the filament
   c. Controls kVp
   d. Is located entirely in the operating console
   e. Is located in all three of the major components of an x-ray imaging system: the console, the high-voltage generator, and the x-ray tube

6. A filament transformer has a turns ratio of 1:20. What current must be supplied to the primary windings if 5 A is required by the filament?
   a. 125 mA
   b. 200 mA
   c. 250 mA
   d. 50 A
   e. 100 A

7. The filament transformer in the previous question is supplied with 150 V to the primary side. What is the secondary voltage?
   a. 750 mV
   b. 3000 mV
   c. 1.5 V
   d. 7.5 V
   e. 30 V

8. The unit mAs:
   a. Could be expressed in coulombs
   b. Could be expressed in meters/second
   c. Is a unit of electric current
   d. Is a unit of electromotive force
   e. Is electrons/second

9. An exposure technique of 100 mA at 100 ms compared with 50 mA at 50 ms results in:
   a. Eight times the total number of electrons
   b. Fewer projectile electrons
   c. Four times the total number of electrons
   d. Three times the total number of electrons
   e. Twice the total number of electrons

10. The control of focal spot size depends on:
   a. The filament that is energized
   b. The mA station selected
   c. The secondary taps of the autotransformer
   d. The target angle selected
   e. The turns ratio of the filament transformer

11. The meter that monitors x-ray tube current is:
    a. Connected to the autotransformer
    b. Connected to the secondary side of the step-down transformer
    c. Grounded to the primary center tap of the step-up transformer
    d. Physically located on the control console
    e. The same as the filament current monitor

12. X-ray tube current is usually measured in which of the following?
    a. Amperes (A)
    b. Ampere-seconds (As)
    c. Microamperes (μA)
    d. Milliamperes (mA)
    e. Milliampere-seconds (mAs)

13. A filament current of 5 A is necessary for thermionic emission. What electron flow is this?
    a. 3.2×10^{15} electrons/s
    b. 3.2×10^{16} electrons/s
    c. 3.2×10^{17} electrons/s
    d. 3.2×10^{18} electrons/s
    e. 3.2×10^{19} electrons/s

14. The filament transformer is designed:
    a. As a step-up transformer
    b. To operate on DC power
    c. With a turns ratio less than 1
    d. With a turns ratio greater than 1
    e. With an mA meter grounded to the center tap

15. Which of the following would be *correct* to use for expressing x-ray tube current?
    a. Coulombs
    b. Meters/second
    c. Electron volts
    d. Kilovolt peak
    e. Kilovolts/second

16. The design of fixed mA stations requires the use of which of the following?
    a. A center-tapped meter
    b. DC power
    c. Major and minor taps
    d. Precision resistors
    e. Primary and secondary windings

17. Operation at 100 mA for 1 s results in which of the following?
    a. 6.3×10^{16} electrons
    b. 6.3×10^{17} electrons/s
    c. 6.3×10^{17} electrons
    d. 6.3×10^{18} electrons/s
    e. 6.3×10^{18} electrons

18. A filament transformer has 800 primary windings and is supplied with 200 mA. If the secondary coil has 100 windings, what will be the secondary current?
    a. 25 mA
    b. 100 mA
    c. 400 mA
    d. 1600 mA
    e. 3200 mA

19. If a filament transformer has a turns ratio of 0.05 and 200 mA is supplied to the primary side of the transformer, what will be the secondary current?
    a. 100 mA
    b. 400 mA
    c. 1 A
    d. 4 A
    e. 6 A

Worksheet 6-3 Operating Console Exposure Timers

Exposure timers are precision devices that start and stop x-ray production. There are four basic types of exposure timers:

1. **Mechanical timers**: These operate by spring action, similarly to a hand-wound alarm clock. These timers are not very accurate, and they are not used on modern equipment.
2. **Synchronous timers**: These timers use a synchronous motor that operates at 60 rpm. Their shortest possible exposure time is 1/60 s.
3. **Electronic timers**: This type of timer operates on an electronic resistive-capacitive circuit based on the time required to charge a capacitor. These timers are accurate, allow exposures as short as 1 millisecond (ms), and can be used for serial radiography.
4. **mAs timers**: These timers are electronic timers that monitor the product of mA and time and terminate the exposure when the proper mAs is reached.

Automatic exposure control (AEC) incorporates a radiation-measuring device that terminates the x-ray exposure when enough x-radiation has reached the image receptor.

EXERCISES

1. A radiographic technique calls for a 50 ms exposure, but the exposure control has only fractional notation. Which of the following should be selected?
   a. 1/60 s
   b. 1/40 s
   c. 1/20 s
   d. 1/10 s
   e. 1/4 s

2. A radiographic technique calls for a 400 mA, 1/20 s exposure. What is the mAs?
   a. 5 mAs
   b. 10 mAs
   c. 20 mAs
   d. 40 mAs
   e. 80 mAs

3. If an x-ray imaging system is operated at 600 mA, 50 ms, the total mAs will be which of the following?
   a. 6 mAs
   b. 30 mAs
   c. 60 mAs
   d. 300 mAs
   e. 600 mAs

4. A radiographic technique of 100 mA at 1/4 s has been used. If one changes to the 500 mA station, the appropriate exposure time for the same mAs is which of the following?
   a. 1/4 s
   b. 3/20 s
   c. 1/20 s
   d. 1/5 s
   e. 1/10 s

5. Operation at 300 mA for 1/20 s is equivalent to operation at 900 mA for:
   a. 8 ms
   b. 17 ms
   c. 60 ms
   d. 200 ms
   e. 500 ms

6. The control of exposure time is always:
   a. Automatically set
   b. Determined by kVp
   c. On the primary side of the autotransformer
   d. On the primary side of the high-voltage transformer
   e. On the secondary side of the filament circuit

7. The exposure timer on a three-phase radiographic imaging system will:
   a. Be automatic
   b. Be electronic
   c. Be synchronous
   d. Limit exposure to 1/60 s or longer
   e. Limit exposure to 8 ms and no shorter

8. An AEC device:
   a. Can use a photomultiplier tube on the entrance side of the patient
   b. Can use an ionization chamber between the patient and the image receptor
   c. Cannot control exposures shorter than $\frac{1}{120}$ s
   d. Does not require a manual timer
   e. Works only with three-phase and high-frequency power

9. With an AEC device:
   a. Exposures less than 100 ms are not possible.
   b. It is not necessary to depress the exposure control.
   c. The exposure starts and stops automatically.
   d. Technique selection is not necessary.
   e. A backup timer is required.

10. The shortest exposure possible with single-phase equipment is $\frac{1}{120}$ s. How many milliseconds is that?
    a. 8 ms
    b. 17 ms
    c. 35 ms
    d. 50 ms
    e. 120 ms

11. Mammography sometimes requires exposures as long as 1.5 s. This is equivalent to which of the following?
    a. 15 ms
    b. 100 ms
    c. 150 ms
    d. 1000 ms
    e. 1500 ms

12. The shortest exposure possible with three-phase equipment is 1 ms. What fraction of a second is that?
    a. $\frac{1}{50}$
    b. $\frac{1}{100}$
    c. $\frac{1}{120}$
    d. $\frac{1}{500}$
    e. $\frac{1}{1000}$

13. There are 30 video frames each second for a fluoroscopic CRT dynamic image. What is the length of each frame?
    a. 1 ms
    b. 10 ms
    c. 16 ms
    d. 33 ms
    e. 60 ms

14. The human eye cannot visualize faster than approximately five views each second. What is the integration time of the human eye?
    a. 1 ms
    b. 10 ms
    c. 20 ms
    d. 100 ms
    e. 200 ms

15. A radiographic technique calls for 86 kVp/200 mAs using the 800 mA station. What is the exposure time?
    a. 10 ms
    b. 25 ms
    c. 100 ms
    d. 250 ms
    e. 500 ms

16. mA is a unit of electric current, and mAs is a unit of:
    a. Electric charge
    b. Electric potential
    c. Reciprocal kVp
    d. X-ray beam quality
    e. X-ray beam quantity

Worksheet 6-4
High-Voltage Generator
High-Voltage Generation

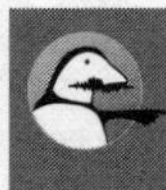

The high-voltage section of the x-ray imaging system contains the following:

- The **high-voltage transformer** ($N_s/N_p > 1$), which converts low voltage from the autotransformer to the required kVp.
- The **filament transformer** ($N_s/N_p > 1$), which reduces the voltage from the autotransformer to about 10 V for heating the filament. At the same time, the filament current is regulated to the range of 4 to 10 A.
- A **rectifier circuit** that converts the alternating voltage into a direct voltage before use by the x-ray tube.

The accompanying figure shows the change in voltage waveform at each stage of generation.

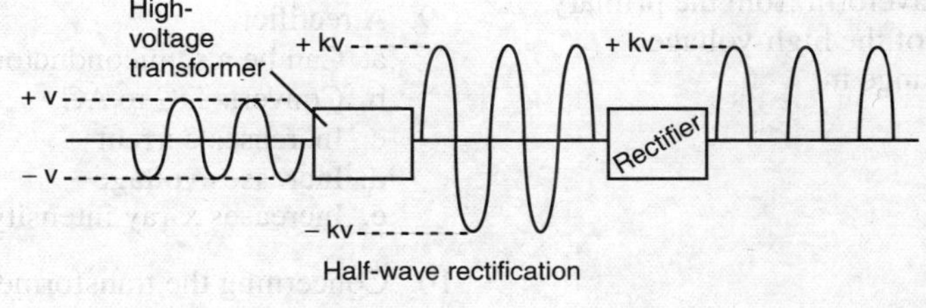

Half-wave rectification

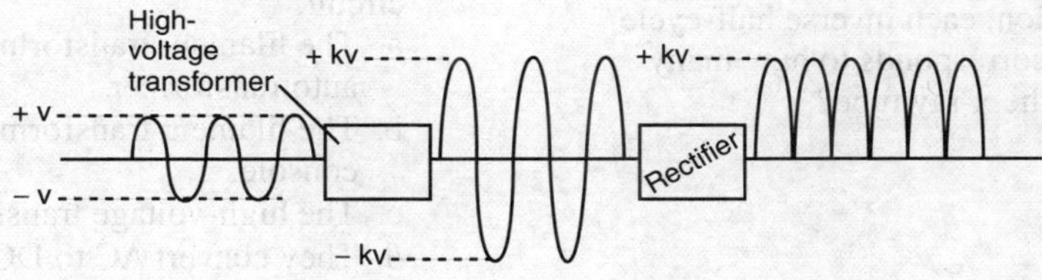

Full-wave rectification

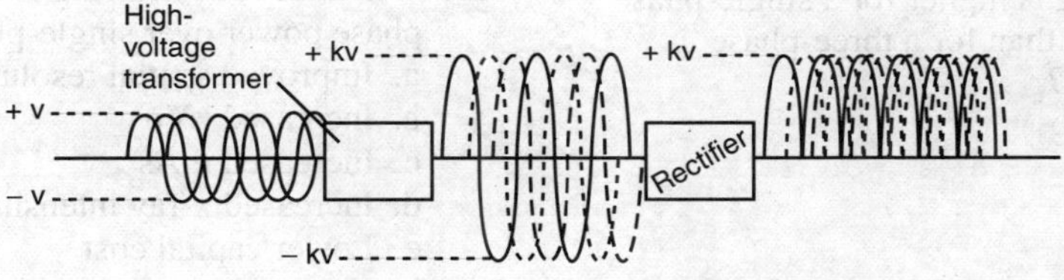

Three-phase rectification

Voltage Waveform	Pulses per Second	Percentage Ripple
Half-wave	60	100
Full-wave	120	100
Three-phase, six-pulse	360	13
Three-phase, 12-pulse	720	4
High frequency	Up to 1000	1

EXERCISES

1. Which of the following is contained in a typical high-voltage generator?
   a. Diode rectifiers
   b. Autotransformer
   c. Exposure switch
   d. kVp meter
   e. mA meter

2. A change in the voltage waveform from the primary side to the secondary side of the high-voltage transformer produces a change in:
   a. Amplitude
   b. Frequency
   c. Phase
   d. Velocity
   e. Wavelength

3. In half-wave rectification, each inverse half-cycle in the primary circuit corresponds to how many voltage pulses across the x-ray tube?
   a. None
   b. One
   c. Two
   d. Four
   e. Twelve

4. Which of the following is higher for a single-phase high-voltage generator than for a three-phase high-voltage generator?
   a. kVp
   b. Purchase price
   c. Rotor speed
   d. Voltage ripple
   e. X-ray quality

5. Which of the following is a disadvantage of three-phase power compared with single-phase power?
   a. Higher capital cost
   b. Higher electrical operating costs
   c. Limited kVp
   d. Longer minimum exposure time
   e. Softer radiation

6. The disadvantage of a self-rectified circuit is:
   a. Its complexity
   b. Its cost
   c. Its limitation of use in dental imaging systems
   d. Its limited exposure time
   e. Its requirement for DC power

7. An exposure of ⅒ s:
   a. At 50 mA is 50 mAs
   b. At 100 mA is 1000 mAs
   c. Is 120 ms
   d. Produces six pulses in full-wave rectification
   e. Produces twice as much radiation if full-wave rectified than if half-wave rectified

8. Full-wave rectification:
   a. Has less ripple compared with half-wave rectification
   b. Is one example of self-rectification
   c. Produces higher kVp than half-wave rectification
   d. Requires at least four rectifiers
   e. Requires at least 12 rectifiers

9. A rectifier:
   a. Can be a semiconductor
   b. Converts DC to AC
   c. Increases current
   d. Increases voltage
   e. Increases x-ray intensity

10. Concerning the transformers used in the x-ray circuit:
    a. The filament transformer is also an autotransformer.
    b. The filament transformer is usually located in the console.
    c. The high-voltage transformer is a step-up device.
    d. They convert AC to DC.
    e. They operate only in DC.

11. Which of the following is an advantage of three-phase power over single-phase power?
    a. Improved spatial resolution
    b. Increased kVp
    c. Increased mAs
    d. Increased x-ray intensity per mAs
    e. Lower capital cost

12. Oil is used in the high-voltage section of an x-ray imaging system for which of the following functions?
    a. Electrical insulation
    b. Reduction of rotor friction
    c. Reduction of voltage ripple
    d. Thermal conduction
    e. Voltage rectification

Worksheet 6-5 High-Voltage Generator Rectification

Nearly everything electric in a hospital operates on alternating current (AC) power. However, in radiology, the most important component of an x-ray imaging system, the x-ray tube, requires direct current (DC).

Circuit elements in the high-voltage generator of the x-ray imaging system, called **rectifiers**, transform the AC to DC. The process of conversion from AC to DC is called **rectification**.

Some types of x-ray imaging systems, primarily dental and portable systems, are capable of transforming AC into DC themselves, while simultaneously producing x-rays. Such a circuit is said to be **self-rectified**. Self-rectification results in half-wave rectification. **Full-wave rectification** is most often used in conventional x-ray imaging systems, and such a circuit requires a minimum of four rectifiers. To full-wave rectify **three-phase power**, a minimum of six rectifiers is required for a six-pulse unit, and 12 are required for a 12-pulse unit.

EXERCISES

1. Which of the following principles of voltage rectification produces the maximum efficiency of x-ray production?
   a. Four-diode rectification
   b. Half-wave rectification
   c. High-frequency generator
   d. Self-rectification
   e. Two-diode rectification

2. To generate three-phase, six-pulse power, at least how many rectifiers are necessary?
   a. 4
   b. 6
   c. 8
   d. 12
   e. 16

3. A semiconductor rectifier:
   a. Has a heated anode
   b. Has a heated cathode
   c. Is a solid-state device
   d. Is an electromechanical device
   e. Is used only for mammography

4. If a single rectifier is inserted into a circuit that conducts 60 Hz AC so that it suppresses the positive portion of the waveform, then the output waveform will contain:
   a. 60 negative pulses per second
   b. 60 positive pulses per second
   c. 120 negative pulses per second
   d. 120 positive pulses per second
   e. Variable pulses, depending on frequency

5. The voltage ripple associated with various x-ray generators is:
   a. 70.7% for single-phase, full-wave rectification
   b. 100% for self-rectification
   c. Higher for self-rectification than for half-wave rectification
   d. Highest with high frequency
   e. Less for single-phase than for three-phase power

6. A rectifier:
   a. Converts AC to DC
   b. Converts DC to AC
   c. Increases voltage
   d. Refers to a type of electromagnetic device
   e. Refers to a type of electromechanical device

7. Near the p-n junction of a semiconductor diode, one will find:
   a. A filtered anode
   b. A heated anode
   c. A heated cathode
   d. A p type of material containing excess electrons
   e. An n type of material containing excess electrons

8. A semiconductor diode:
   a. Allows current to flow only from n type of material to p type
   b. Allows current to flow only from p type of material to n type
   c. Contains carriers that are also called proton traps
   d. Contains holes that are also called proton traps
   e. Is also called an electromechanical rectifier

9. In a circuit that contains a single rectifier:
   a. Electron flow is pulsed but uninterrupted.
   b. Electrons flow in one direction but not the other.
   c. The result is constant potential DC.
   d. Twice as many electrons flow in the output coil as in the input coil.
   e. Voltage is increased.

10. If 60 Hz AC power is full-wave rectified, output voltage consists of:
   a. 60 pulses per second
   b. 90 pulses per second
   c. 120 pulses per second
   d. 70% ripple
   e. Zero ripple

11. The current from a common household wall receptacle in the United States is:
   a. 50 Hz AC
   b. 50 Hz DC
   c. 60 Hz AC
   d. 60 Hz DC
   e. Constant potential

12. Thermionic emission refers to:
   a. Electron emission from a heated source
   b. Heat conduction
   c. Heat emission from an electric conductor
   d. Heat radiation
   e. Ionization with heat

13. The main advantage of full-wave rectification over half-wave rectification is:
   a. Higher-energy x-rays
   b. Higher kVp
   c. Higher mA
   d. Less voltage ripple
   e. A greater number of x-rays per cycle

14. How many overlapping pulses are generated in 1 s for three-phase, six-pulse power?
   a. 60
   b. 120
   c. 360
   d. 720
   e. 2160

Match the approximate voltage ripple with each of the following. Some answers may be used more than once.

______ 15. Full-wave rectified	a. 1%
______ 16. High frequency	b. 4%
______ 17. Three-phase, six-pulse	c. 14%
______ 18. Three-phase, 12-pulse	d. 75%
______ 19. Self-rectified	e. 100%

Worksheet 7-1
Internal Components
The X-Ray Tube Cathode

The cathode is the negative side of the x-ray tube. Its major components are the **filament** and the **focusing cup**. The filament is a small coil of wire, usually of thoriated tungsten, that provides electrons for the production of x-rays. The focusing cup directs the beam of electrons to the target on the anode.

Tungsten vaporization with deposition on the inside of a glass enclosure x-ray tube is the most common cause of x-ray tube failure.

EXERCISES

1. The three principal parts of an x-ray imaging system are:
   a. Anode, cathode, and focusing cup
   b. Anode, cathode, and high-voltage generator
   c. X-ray tube, control console, and high-voltage generator
   d. X-ray tube, high-voltage generator, and image receptor
   e. X-ray tube, protective housing, and high-voltage generator

2. The primary purpose of the glass envelope of an x-ray tube is to:
   a. Control leakage radiation
   b. Control off-focus radiation
   c. Cool the tube
   d. Ensure against electric shock
   e. Provide a vacuum

3. The protective housing of an x-ray tube is designed to:
   a. Control isotropic x-ray emission
   b. Control scatter radiation
   c. Limit operation to 100 kVp or less
   d. Reduce the hazard of leakage radiation
   e. Reduce the hazard of scatter radiation

4. A diagnostic x-ray tube is an example of which of the following?
   a. Cathode
   b. Diode
   c. Tetrode
   d. Anode
   e. Electrode

5. The large filament is used during radiography when the heat load is:
   a. High, and visibility of detail is important
   b. High, and visibility of detail is less important
   c. Low, and high kVp is required
   d. Low, and visibility of detail is important
   e. Low, and visibility of detail is less important

6. In most x-ray tubes, there are two filaments to:
   a. Ensure saturation current
   b. Produce higher-energy x-rays
   c. Provide two electrodes
   d. Provide two focal spots
   e. Reduce space charge effects

7. The focusing cup:
   a. Is on the positive side of the x-ray tube
   b. Is slightly positive with respect to the filament
   c. Is the grid in a grid-controlled x-ray tube
   d. Is usually made of thoriated tungsten
   e. Selects the filament

8. Once filament temperature becomes adequate, a further small rise in filament temperature will cause tube current to:
   a. Decrease just a bit
   b. Decrease very much
   c. Increase just a bit
   d. Increase very much
   e. Not change

9. The cathode beam of an x-ray tube is the:
   a. Current that heats the filament
   b. Focused electron beam within the tube
   c. Off-focus radiation
   d. Primary x-ray beam
   e. Secondary radiation

10. The x-ray tube current:
   a. Controls x-ray energy
   b. Flows through both filaments at the same time
   c. Is controlled by the filament current
   d. Is the current that flows through the filament
   e. Usually varies from 50 to 1000 A

11. Most x-ray tubes used for radiography:
    a. Are dual-focus tubes
    b. Do not emit leakage radiation
    c. Have a fixed anode
    d. Operate in the space charge–limited mode
    e. Use tungsten filaments that do not vaporize

12. The cathode is:
    a. A diode
    b. Designed to supply heat
    c. One of the two parts of a diode
    d. Part of the target
    e. Positively charged

13. When a filament burns out:
    a. It should be replaced within 30 days.
    b. The filament current goes to maximum.
    c. The filament current goes to zero.
    d. The tube current is maximum.
    e. The x-ray intensity is maximum.

14. The space charge effect:
    a. Is more pronounced at high kVp
    b. Is more pronounced at low mA
    c. Limits kVp
    d. Occurs in the vicinity of the anode
    e. Occurs in the vicinity of the cathode

15. The x-ray tube filament:
    a. Conducts approximately 5 A
    b. Conducts current only when an exposure is made
    c. Is a diode
    d. Is the space charge
    e. Is usually copper

16. If saturation is achieved and the filament current is fixed, tube current:
    a. Decreases with use
    b. Falls with increasing kVp
    c. Remains fixed
    d. Rises with increasing exposure time
    e. Rises with increasing kVp

17. X-ray tube current:
    a. Depends on exposure time
    b. Depends on voltage
    c. Increases when the kVp is decreased
    d. Is measured in milliamperes rather than amperes
    e. Is zero when filament current is below thermionic emission

Worksheet 7-2
Internal Components
The X-Ray Tube Anode

The x-ray tube anode serves four principal functions: (1) **electrical conduction** of the x-ray tube current, (2) **mechanical support** for the target, (3) **thermal conduction** of heat, and (4) **x-ray production**. The active portion of the anode, in which x-rays are produced, is the target. Almost all targets are made of tungsten (usually alloyed with rhenium). However, some used exclusively for mammography have molybdenum or rhodium targets.

The area of the target on which the projectile electrons interact is the **focal spot**. All diagnostic x-ray tubes have an inclined anode to exploit the **line-focus principle**.

Tungsten is the element of choice for the target for general radiography for three main reasons: atomic number (Z = 74), thermal conductivity, and high melting point.

EXERCISES

1. A stationary-anode x-ray tube:
   a. Incorporates the line-focus principle
   b. Is used to produce very short exposures
   c. Limits leakage radiation
   d. Provides for greater heat dissipation
   e. Usually has a very small focal spot

2. The heel effect occurs because of:
   a. A focusing cup
   b. Reduced tube current
   c. The shape charge effect
   d. The shape of the filament
   e. X-ray absorption in the anode

3. The main reason for using the line-focus principle is to:
   a. Increase heat capacity
   b. Increase x-ray intensity
   c. Reduce exposure time
   d. Reduce focal-spot size
   e. Reduce heel effect

4. Rotating anode x-ray tubes:
   a. Have a copper target embedded in a tungsten anode
   b. Have a tungsten target embedded in a copper anode
   c. Have target angles that are less than 10 degrees
   d. Incorporate the line-focus principle
   e. Produce higher-energy x-rays

5. X-ray intensity is higher on the cathode side than on the anode side because of which of the following?
   a. The focusing cup
   b. The line-focus principle
   c. The space charge effect
   d. X-ray absorption in the anode
   e. X-ray deflection from the anode

6. Which of the following target angles is characteristic of a rotating anode x-ray tube?
   a. 1 degree
   b. 20 degrees
   c. 25 degrees
   d. 50 degrees
   e. 100 degrees

7. Small target angles result in which of the following?
   a. Better collimation
   b. Increased heat capacity
   c. Less heel effect
   d. Small focal-spot size
   e. Small space charge

8. Molybdenum is used for anode stem material because of which of the following?
   a. It has a high atomic number.
   b. It has a shiny surface and reflects electrons well.
   c. It has a longer life.
   d. It is a good heat conductor.
   e. It is a poor thermal conductor.

9. Tungsten is the choice material for x-ray anodes because of its:
   a. High atomic number
   b. High rpm
   c. High x-ray intensity
   d. Low atomic number
   e. Low rpm

10. The effective focal spot is:
    a. Larger than the actual focal spot
    b. Largest on the anode side of the central axis
    c. Smaller than the actual focal spot
    d. Smallest on the cathode side of the central axis
    e. The same size as the actual focal spot

11. The heel effect:
    a. Is more pronounced when large target angles are used
    b. Is reduced with a focusing cup
    c. Occurs only with rotating anode x-ray tubes
    d. Requires that the cathode be positioned to the thicker anatomy
    e. Suggests that the cathode be up during posteroanterior chest radiography

12. What is a prominent engineering difficulty in the manufacture of high-speed rotating anodes?
    a. Balance of the rotor
    b. Control of space charge effects
    c. Marriage to the focusing cup
    d. Proper target angle
    e. Target-face polish

13. Which of the following is a component of an electromagnetic induction motor?
    a. Cathode
    b. Filament
    c. Stator
    d. Target angle
    e. Target disc

14. Necessary properties of x-ray target material include which of the following?
    a. High melting point
    b. High rotation speed
    c. Low atomic number
    d. Low coefficient of friction
    e. High electrical resistance

15. Which of the following is an advantage of the rotating anode tube over the stationary anode tube?
    a. Higher heat capacity
    b. Higher kVp capacity
    c. Longer exposure time
    d. Reduced heel effect
    e. The line-focus principle

16. The anode angle of an x-ray tube is increased to give which of the following?
    a. Smaller focal spot
    b. Higher heat capacity
    c. Proper focusing of the electron beam
    d. Proper reflection
    e. Uniform x-ray intensity

17. Which of the following components of a diagnostic x-ray tube is on the positive side of the tube?
    a. The cathode
    b. The filament
    c. The focusing cup
    d. The grid
    e. The stator

18. As the anode target angle increases:
    a. Effective focal-spot size increases.
    b. Heel effect becomes more pronounced.
    c. kVp increases.
    d. Radiation intensity on the central ray increases.
    e. Target rotating speed increases.

19. A stationary anode will *most* likely be used in which of the following?
    a. Chest radiography
    b. Dentistry
    c. General radiography
    d. Interventional radiology
    e. Mammography

20. Which of the following is *not* a function of the anode?
    a. Conduction of electricity
    b. Mechanical support
    c. Thermal conduction
    d. Thermionic emission
    e. X-ray production

21. Which of the following is the principal hurdle in the design of an x-ray anode for high-capacity radiologic techniques?
    a. Heat dissipation
    b. Radiation quality
    c. Radiation quantity
    d. Rotating speed
    e. X-ray intensity

Worksheet 7-3
X-Ray Tube Failure
X-Ray Tube Rating Charts

The three types of tube rating charts are the radiographic rating chart, the anode cooling chart, and the housing cooling chart.

The **radiographic rating chart** shows which single radiographic techniques are within the safe limits of operation for a particular x-ray tube. The **anode cooling chart** displays the thermal capacity of the anode and the time required for the heated anode to cool. The **housing cooling chart** gives the maximum heat capacity of the x-ray tube housing, as well as the time required for that housing to cool. Thermal energy absorbed by the anode is measured in **heat units (HU)**.

$$1\ \text{J} = 1\ \text{kV} \times 1\ \text{mA} \times 1\ \text{s}$$

$$1\ \text{HU} = \text{kVp} \times \text{mA} \times \text{Second for single-phase power} = 0.7\ \text{J}$$

$$1\ \text{HU} = 1.4\ \text{kVp} \times \text{mA} \times \text{Seconds for three-phase and high-frequency power}$$

$$1\ \text{HU} = 1.4\ \text{J for three-phase and high-frequency power}$$

EXERCISES

1. If the intersection of time and kVp falls on an mA curve, that mA is safe.
   a. True
   b. False

2. Most of the troublesome heat generated in an x-ray tube occurs at the filament.
   a. True
   b. False

3. Generally, a larger focal spot allows longer exposure times than a smaller focal spot.
   a. True
   b. False

4. The anode cooling chart reports the time that should elapse between exposures.
   a. True
   b. False

5. It is *not* possible to exceed the heat capacity of the housing without first exceeding that of the anode.
   a. True
   b. False

6. A tube can become “gassy” because of anode overheating and the release of gas.
   a. True
   b. False

7. The radiographic rating chart is designed primarily to protect the filament.
   a. True
   b. False

8. Rotor speed does influence heat capacity.
   a. True
   b. False

9. HU can be expressed as exposure rate in Gy_a/min.
   a. True
   b. False

10. How many heat units are produced by the following radiographic technique? 100 kVp, 150 mA, 500 ms, single phase, 3400 rpm, 0.6 mm focal spot.

11. To determine whether any set of tube rating charts is applicable for a given x-ray tube, one should:
    a. Check to see that the operating console will allow operation at 150 kVp because this is the maximum indicated on all radiographic rating charts.
    b. Determine whether the operating console allows all of the mA settings indicated for the radiographic rating chart.
    c. Identify the type of tube, the anode rotation, the focal-spot size, and the type of generator to make certain that all of these match the specifications on the chart.
    d. Make an exposure at a radiographic technique that exceeds the maximum permitted by the charts, and check to see whether the interlock circuit prevents the exposure.
    e. Warm the tube with five rapid exposures.

12. If a single exposure were made with factors *slightly* exceeding those permitted by the appropriate radiographic rating chart, which of the following would be the *most* probable result?
    a. The anode would pit or crack.
    b. The glass envelope would crack.
    c. The rotor would freeze and stop.
    d. The tube filament would burn out.
    e. The useful life of the tube would be reduced.

13. If a single exposure were made with factors *greatly* exceeding those permitted by the appropriate radiographic rating chart, which of the following would be the *most* probable result?
    a. The anode would pit or crack.
    b. The glass envelope would crack.
    c. The rotor would freeze and stop.
    d. The tube filament would break.
    e. The tube would become gassy.

14. Which of the following conditions will *not* damage an x-ray tube?
    a. Exceeding the anode heat storage capacity
    b. Exceeding the heat storage capacity of the tube housing
    c. Exceeding the instantaneous filament emission rate
    d. Exceeding the prescribed source-to-image receptor distance
    e. Successive high-intensity exposures

15. In the design of a rotating anode x-ray tube:
    a. Dual-focus tubes require two high-voltage, step-up transformers.
    b. Dual-focus tubes require two separate anodes.
    c. Dual-focus tubes require two target materials.
    d. Most anodes rotate at 3400 or 10,000 rpm.
    e. The disc can be made thicker so that the rpm can be increased.

16. A fluoroscopic examination at 85 kVp and 4 mA, single phase, requires 4 min. The number of anode heat units produced would be approximately:
    a. 1360
    b. 1836
    c. 40,800
    d. 81,600
    e. 96,400

17. The formula for HU in a single-phase high-voltage generator is:
    a. kVp × mA × s
    b. kVp × mA × s^2
    c. kVp × mAs × s
    d. kVp × mAs × s^2
    e. kVp × mA × s^{-1}

Worksheet 8-1 Electron-Target Interactions Characteristic Radiation

In characteristic x-ray production, the projectile electron ionizes a target atom by removing a tightly bound inner-shell electron. The hole created in the inner electron shell of the target atom is filled by an outer-shell electron or a free electron falling into the hole. This transition of an electron from an outer shell to an inner shell is accompanied by the emission of an x-ray of energy equal to the difference between the binding energies of the two electron shells involved. For example, if a K-shell electron is ejected and replaced with an L-shell electron, a characteristic x-ray with energy as calculated below will be released.

Energy of characteristic x-ray =
BE_K shell electron – BE_L shell electron
(Binding energy of ejected electron) (Binding energy of ejected electron)

Approximate Electron-Binding Energy, keV

Shell	Molybdenum (Mo)	Tungsten (W)
K	20.0	69.0
L	3.0	12.0
M	0.5	2.0
N	—	1.0
O	—	0.1

EXERCISES

1. If mass is expressed in kilograms and velocity in meters per second, kinetic energy will be expressed in:
   a. Coulombs
   b. Electron volts
   c. Ergs
   d. Joules
   e. Newtons

2. The kinetic energy of the projectile electron in an x-ray tube:
   a. Causes excitation in the vacuum of the x-ray tube
   b. Causes ionization in the vacuum of the x-ray tube
   c. Is about 1% efficient in the production of x-rays
   d. Is converted to mass
   e. Is totally converted to x-ray energy

3. The shift of the characteristic x-ray spectrum to higher energy occurs because of which of the following?
   a. A decrease in voltage ripple
   b. A decrease in kVp
   c. A higher atomic number filter
   d. An increase in kVp
   e. An increase in target atomic number

4. Useful characteristic x-rays are produced in tungsten:
   a. By excitation of a K-shell electron
   b. By removal of a K-shell electron
   c. By ionization of an L-shell electron
   d. When a valence electron is removed
   e. When the projectile electron interacts with an outer-shell electron

5. An L-shell electron (binding energy 26 keV) is removed from an atom that has M-shell binding energy of 4 keV and N-shell binding energy of 1 keV. If a free electron fills the vacancy in the L-shell, the characteristic x-ray produced will have an energy of:
   a. 1 keV
   b. 4 keV
   c. 22 keV
   d. 25 keV
   e. 26 keV

6. What is produced when the projectile electron excites an outer-shell electron?
   a. Bremsstrahlung x-ray
   b. Characteristic x-ray
   c. Energy
   d. Heat
   e. Photoelectric x-ray

7. The energy of characteristic x-rays increases with increasing:
   a. Filtration
   b. Atomic mass of a target material
   c. Atomic number of a target material
   d. kVp
   e. Voltage waveform

8. X-rays are produced when:
   a. Electric current flows through the x-ray tube filament.
   b. Projectile electrons bounce off the cathode.
   c. Projectile electrons interact with target atoms.
   d. The target angle is sufficiently large.
   e. The x-ray tube filament is heated to thermionic emission.

9. Characteristic x-rays:
   a. Are characteristic of target Z
   b. Are characteristic of the filter material
   c. Are characteristic of the voltage waveform
   d. Have velocity varying from zero to the speed of light
   e. Vary in energy as kVp is varied

10. When a tungsten-targeted x-ray tube is operated at 68 kVp:
    a. K-shell characteristic x-rays can be produced.
    b. L-shell x-rays cannot be produced.
    c. One possible K-shell characteristic x-ray will have 12 keV of energy.
    d. Some projectile electrons may have 68 keV of energy.
    e. Some projectile electrons may have 75 keV of energy.

11. According to the table above:
    a. The farther from the nucleus, the higher the electron-binding energy.
    b. The K-shell characteristic x-rays of molybdenum are lower in energy than the L-shell characteristic x-rays of tungsten.
    c. The L-shell characteristic x-rays of molybdenum are of higher energy than the L-shell characteristic x-rays of tungsten.
    d. Tungsten obviously has a lower atomic number than molybdenum.
    e. Tungsten obviously has a greater number of electrons than molybdenum.

12. When characteristic x-rays are produced, the energy of the x-rays is characteristic of:
    a. The atomic number of the filter
    b. The atomic number of the target
    c. The outer-shell electron-binding energy
    d. The mass of filtration
    e. The orientation of the target

13. Gold is sometimes used as a target material in special types of radiation-producing systems. Its electron-binding energies are as follows: K-shell: 81 keV; L-shell: 14 keV; M-shell: 3 keV; and N-shell: 1 keV. Which of the following characteristic x-rays would be produced with operation at 90 kVp?
    a. 12 keV
    b. 67 keV
    c. 76 keV
    d. 87 keV
    e. 90 keV

14. The kinetic energy of a projectile electron can be measured in:
    a. Amperes
    b. Coulombs
    c. Joules
    d. Newtons
    e. Watts

15. The efficiency of x-ray production is:
    a. Approximately 5%
    b. Greater than that of heat production
    c. In excess of 5%
    d. Independent of tube current
    e. Independent of tube voltage

16. The joules (J) of energy generated by electron-target interactions are given by:
    a. kV × mA × s
    b. kV × mA × ms
    c. kVp × mA × s
    d. kVp × mA × s × s
    e. kVp × mA × ms

Worksheet 8-2
Electron-Target Interactions
Bremsstrahlung Radiation

Bremsstrahlung x-rays are produced when a projectile electron from the cathode passes close enough to the nucleus to be influenced by the nucleus. As the projectile electron passes the nucleus, the electron slows and its direction changes. Therefore it leaves the electron with reduced kinetic energy.

The loss in kinetic energy reappears as an x-ray. These are bremsstrahlung x-rays. They can have energy ranging from zero to a maximum that is equal to the projectile electron energy. The most frequent bremsstrahlung x-ray energy is approximately one-third of the maximum energy of the projectile electron. Most x-rays in a diagnostic x-ray beam are bremsstrahlung x-rays.

EXERCISES

1. In a tungsten-targeted x-ray tube operated at 90 kVp, the *most* abundant x-ray would be a:
   a. 10 keV characteristic x-ray
   b. 12 keV characteristic x-ray
   c. 30 keV bremsstrahlung x-ray
   d. 69 keV bremsstrahlung x-ray
   e. 90 keV bremsstrahlung x-ray

2. Which of the following electron transitions results in the *most* useful bremsstrahlung x-ray?
   a. L to K
   b. M to K
   c. M to L
   d. O to K
   e. None of the above

3. Bremsstrahlung radiation is produced by:
   a. Conversion of projectile electron kinetic energy to electromagnetic energy
   b. Conversion of target electron kinetic energy to electromagnetic energy
   c. Intrashell electron transitions
   d. Projectile electron-target electron interaction
   e. Target electron-nuclear interaction

4. When a bremsstrahlung x-ray is produced:
   a. A projectile electron is absorbed.
   b. A projectile electron loses energy.
   c. A target electron is displaced.
   d. A target electron is excited.
   e. A target electron is ionized.

5. In bremsstrahlung x-ray production:
   a. The projectile electron is bound to tungsten.
   b. The projectile electron is from the cathode.
   c. The target electron exists as a free electron.
   d. The target electron is from the cathode.
   e. The target electron is ionized.

6. If an average radiographic technique is used:
   a. Excitation of the target is approximately 50%.
   b. Ionization of the target is almost complete.
   c. Maximum-energy x-ray is the electron-binding energy.
   d. Most x-rays are bremsstrahlung.
   e. Most x-rays are characteristic.

7. Bremsstrahlung x-rays are produced only at:
   a. Discrete energies
   b. Energies above characteristic x-rays
   c. Energies below characteristic x-rays
   d. Energies up to projectile electron energy
   e. Projectile electron kinetic energy

8. If radiographic technique is 74 kVp/80 mAs:
   a. Bremsstrahlung x-ray energy increases if the voltage is increased to 84 kVp.
   b. Bremsstrahlung x-rays are emitted at discrete energies.
   c. Bremsstrahlung x-rays have a maximum energy of 80 keV.
   d. Characteristic x-ray energy increases if the voltage is increased to 84 kVp.
   e. Characteristic x-rays are emitted only at 74 keV.

9. If radiographic technique in a tungsten target at 60 kVp/80 mAs is changed to 80 kVp/80 mAs:
   a. Additional filtration is required.
   b. Bremsstrahlung x-ray intensity remains unchanged.
   c. Characteristic x-ray intensity remains unchanged.
   d. The number of projectile electrons increases.
   e. The number of x-rays produced increases.

10. Bremsstrahlung x-rays produced in a tungsten-targeted x-ray tube:
    a. Are all diagnostically useful
    b. Are generally less useful than characteristic x-rays
    c. Are less intense than characteristic x-rays
    d. Are less intense than if produced in molybdenum
    e. Outnumber characteristic x-rays

11. When a bremsstrahlung x-ray is emitted:
    a. A projectile electron is absorbed.
    b. An inner-shell electron is removed from the target atom.
    c. An outer-shell electron is removed from the target atom.
    d. This results from the conversion of kinetic energy.
    e. The target atom is ionized.

12. The wavelength of an x-ray:
    a. Becomes longer as projectile electron kinetic energy is reduced
    b. Becomes longer with increasing projectile electron energy
    c. Is longer than that of ultraviolet light
    d. Is longest when the projectile electron loses all its kinetic energy
    e. Is proportional to its frequency

13. When projectile electron energy is increased:
    a. Characteristic x-ray energy decreases.
    b. Characteristic x-ray energy increases.
    c. More bremsstrahlung x-rays are produced.
    d. More bremsstrahlung x-rays are produced, but only at high energies.
    e. More bremsstrahlung x-rays are produced, but only at low energies.

14. The efficiency of bremsstrahlung x-ray production increases with increasing:
    a. Collimation
    b. Filtration
    c. mA
    d. source-to-image receptor distance
    e. Target atomic number

15. The output intensity of an x-ray tube:
    a. Increases when filtered
    b. Is limited by the K-shell binding energy
    c. Is monoenergetic
    d. Often is measured in curies (becquerels)
    e. Is primarily due to bremsstrahlung x-rays

16. Which of the following projectile electron-target interactions results in x-ray emission?
    a. Excitation of inner-shell electron
    b. Excitation of outer-shell electron
    c. Removal of inner-shell electron
    d. Removal of nucleus
    e. Removal of outer-shell electron

17. When a projectile electron enters a target atom and interacts with the nuclear force field:
    a. It decreases in velocity.
    b. It increases in velocity.
    c. It ionizes the atom.
    d. It ionizes the nucleus.
    e. It removes an inner-shell electron.

18. In a tungsten-targeted x-ray tube operated at 90 kVp, the most abundant x-ray would be a:
    a. 10 keV characteristic x-ray
    b. 12 keV characteristic x-ray
    c. 30 keV bremsstrahlung x-ray
    d. 69 keV bremsstrahlung x-ray
    e. 90 keV bremsstrahlung x-ray

Worksheet 8-3
X-Ray Emission Spectrum

An x-ray emission spectrum is a graph of the relative number of x-rays plotted as a function of the energy of each x-ray.

The characteristic x-ray emission spectrum represents monoenergetic x-rays emitted after ionization of the target atom. It consists of vertical lines at fixed energies and is called a **discrete** x-ray emission spectrum.

The bremsstrahlung x-ray emission spectrum results from x-rays created by the bremsstrahlung process and has energy ranging from zero to the maximum projectile electron energy. This spectrum is the **continuous** emission spectrum, and its maximum amplitude occurs at an energy that is approximately one-third of the maximum energy.

EXERCISES

1. The area under the curve of the x-ray emission spectrum represents:
   a. The average energy of the x-rays
   b. The average number of x-rays per unit of energy
   c. The total energy of the x-rays
   d. The total number of x-rays
   e. Total exposure (mGy_a)

2. Normally, the x-ray emission spectrum contains:
   a. Both characteristic and bremsstrahlung x-rays
   b. Both photoelectric and Compton x-rays
   c. Only bremsstrahlung x-rays
   d. Only characteristic x-rays
   e. Only discrete lines

3. The characteristic x-ray emission spectrum principally depends on which of the following?
   a. Filtration
   b. kVp
   c. mAs
   d. Projectile electron energy
   e. Target material

4. The continuous x-ray emission spectrum principally depends on which of the following?
   a. Exposure time
   b. Filtration
   c. mAs
   d. Projectile electron energy
   e. Target material

5. Which of the following factors explains the low number of x-rays emitted at low energy?
   a. Added filtration
   b. The glass envelope of the x-ray tube
   c. The kVp
   d. The mAs enclosing the x-ray tube
   e. The product of tube current and exposure time

6. The x-ray emission spectrum represents:
   a. Projectile electron energy
   b. Atomic mass and number of the target atom
   c. Electron-binding energy of target material
   d. Total x-ray beam filtration
   e. X-rays emitted from the x-ray tube

7. Both the shape and the position of the characteristic x-ray emission spectrum:
   a. Are described by the number of projectile electrons
   b. Represent projectile electron energy
   c. Can be described as continuous
   d. Correspond to target electron-binding energies
   e. Result from nuclear interaction

8. A diagnostic x-ray beam contains:
   a. Bremsstrahlung only
   b. Mostly bremsstrahlung x-rays, with some characteristic x-rays
   c. Mostly Compton x-rays, few bremsstrahlung x-rays, and some pair production x-rays
   d. Some Compton x-rays, some bremsstrahlung x-rays, and no pair production x-rays
   e. Some photoelectric x-rays

9. The x-ray emission spectrum is a plot of:
   a. mAs versus kVp
   b. The number of electrons versus energy
   c. The number of x-rays versus energy
   d. X-rays and electrons emitted from cathode atoms
   e. X-rays and electrons emitted from target atoms

10. The amplitude of the bremsstrahlung x-ray emission spectrum:
    a. Approaches maximum at an energy equal to the kVp
    b. Approaches maximum at zero energy
    c. Has maximum value at energy approximately one-third of the kVp
    d. Has maximum value at an energy equal to the kVp
    e. Is enhanced with filtration

11. If an x-ray emission spectrum represented operation at 85 kVp with a tungsten target:
    a. At 85 keV, the number of projectile electrons would be maximum.
    b. Bremsstrahlung x-rays would be most intense at 85 keV.
    c. The K-characteristic x-ray emission would occur at 69 keV.
    d. X-rays representing maximum frequency would occur at 69 keV.
    e. X-rays representing minimum wavelength would occur at 0 keV.

12. If an x-ray emission spectrum represented operation at 26 kVp with a molybdenum target:
    a. K-characteristic x-rays would not be produced.
    b. More characteristic bremsstrahlung x-rays would be emitted.
    c. The characteristic radiation would have an energy of approximately 19 keV.
    d. Maximum-frequency x-rays would have an energy of 17 keV.
    e. Minimum-wavelength x-rays would have an energy of 20 keV.

13. Which of the following factors principally accounts for the reduced x-ray intensity at low energy?
    a. Added filtration
    b. Beam collimation
    c. Atomic number of the target material
    d. Energy spectrum of the projectile electrons
    e. Voltage waveform

14. Characteristic x-radiation is related to the:
    a. Difference between K- and L-shell binding energy
    b. Energy required to eject K-shell electrons
    c. Energy to eject L-shell electrons
    d. Number of electrons
    e. Number of K-shell electrons

15. Molybdenum has a lower atomic number than tungsten; therefore the molybdenum x-ray emission spectrum:
    a. Extends to higher energies
    b. Extends to lower energies
    c. Has higher amplitude
    d. Has higher-energy characteristic x-rays
    e. Has lower amplitude

16. To construct an x-ray emission spectrum, one must know the:
    a. kVp and mAs
    b. mAs and x-ray frequency
    c. Number of x-rays at each energy interval
    d. Projectile electron number and energy interval
    e. Target element and filtration

Worksheet 8-4
X-Ray Emission Spectrum Minimum Wavelength

X-ray emission sometimes is shown as a function of x-ray wavelength rather than energy. Because x-ray energy and wavelength are inversely proportional, the highest x-ray energy corresponds to the shortest x-ray wavelength, which is also called the **minimum wavelength**.

Planck quantum equation is:

$$E = hf$$

where

$$f = \frac{c}{\lambda}$$

Therefore:

$$E = \frac{hc}{\lambda}$$

$$E = \frac{(4.14 \times 10^{-15}\ \text{eVs})\ (3 \times 10^{8}\ \text{m/s})}{\lambda}$$

$$E = \frac{12.4 \times 10^{-7}\ \text{eVm}}{\lambda}\ \frac{1\ \text{keV}}{10^{3}\ \text{eV}}$$

$$E = \frac{12.4 \times 10^{-10}\ \text{keVm}}{\lambda}$$

This equation can be rearranged to solve for λ, which is the wavelength of an x-ray having energy E in keV:

$$\lambda = \frac{12.4 \times 10^{-10}\ \text{keV m}}{E}$$

$$\lambda_{min} = \frac{12.4 \times 10^{-10}\ \text{keV m}}{\text{kVp}}$$

$$\lambda_{min}(\text{nm}) = \frac{1.24}{\text{kVp}}$$

EXERCISES

1. Which characteristic is reduced as x-ray energy increases?
   a. Filtration
   b. Projectile electron energy
   c. Target electron energy
   d. X-ray frequency
   e. X-ray wavelength

2. The wavelength of an x-ray is:
   a. Determined by filter thickness
   b. Determined by the number of projectile electrons
   c. Determined by the number of target electrons
   d. Directly proportional to its energy
   e. Inversely proportional to its energy

3. The product of Planck constant (h) and the velocity of light (c) has units of:
   a. Jm^2
   b. Jm
   c. J/m
   d. Js
   e. J/s

4. The product of Planck constant (h) and the velocity of light (c) equals:
   a. 12.4 eVm
   b. 12.4 keVm
   c. 12.4×10^{-7} eVm
   d. 12.4×10^{-10} eVm
   e. 12.4×10^{-15} eVm

5. If one knows the minimum wavelength of a given x-ray beam, the kVp of operation can be determined if one also knows which of the following fixed values?
   a. Planck constant
   b. Nothing more is needed
   c. The mA
   d. The mAs
   e. The voltage waveform

6. Minimum wavelength is related to:
   a. Nuclear charge
   b. The atomic number of the target material
   c. The degree of collimation of the x-ray beam
   d. The kinetic energy of the projectile electron
   e. The total filtration in the x-ray beam

7. That region of the x-ray emission spectrum associated with minimum wavelength is the:
   a. Highest-energy bremsstrahlung x-ray
   b. Highest-energy characteristic line
   c. Intersection of the two axes
   d. Lowest-energy bremsstrahlung x-ray
   e. Lowest-energy characteristic line

8. If one knows the minimum wavelength of an x-ray emission spectrum, one can calculate:
   a. Filter atomic number
   b. Filtration thickness
   c. mA
   d. mAs
   e. Maximum projectile electron energy

9. To calculate the minimum x-ray wavelength, one must know the value of:
   a. Filtration
   b. kVp
   c. mA
   d. mAs
   e. Phase

10. How would the total emission spectrum be affected if the x-ray technique changed from 80 kVp and 80 mAs to 80 kVp/400 mA/100 ms? The relative position of the spectrum would:
    a. Remain the same
    b. Remain the same, but the amplitude would decrease
    c. Remain the same, but the amplitude would increase
    d. Shift to the left, and the amplitude would be lower
    e. Shift to the right

11. How would the emission spectrum be affected by the addition of 2 mm Al filtration? The relative position of the spectrum would:
    a. Remain the same
    b. Remain the same, but the amplitude would decrease
    c. Remain the same, but the amplitude would increase
    d. Shift to the left and the amplitude would be lower
    e. Shift to the right and the amplitude would be lower

12. How would the emission spectrum be affected if the power supply were changed from single phase to three phase? The relative position of the spectrum would:
    a. Not change, but the energy of the characteristic lines would increase.
    b. Remain the same.
    c. Remain the same, the amplitude would increase, and the characteristic lines would increase in height.
    d. Shift to the left, the amplitude would increase, and the characteristic lines would increase in height.
    e. Shift to the right, the amplitude would increase, and the characteristic lines would increase in height.

Worksheet 8-5
X-Ray Emission Spectrum
Factors That Affect the X-Ray Emission Spectrum

The shape of the emission spectrum and its relative position vary with changes in kVp, mAs, filtration, target material, and voltage waveform. Higher amplitude in the emission spectrum represents greater x-ray intensity (beam quantity), whereas a shift of the spectrum to the right along the energy axis represents greater penetrability (beam quality).

In general, the following relationships apply:

- Increasing kVp increases the height of the x-ray emission spectrum and extends it to the right along the energy axis.
- Increasing mAs increases the height of the x-ray emission spectrum.
- Increasing filtration decreases the height of the x-ray emission spectrum and shifts the shape to the right along the energy axis.
- Changing to a higher atomic number x-ray target increases the x-ray emission spectrum amplitude, shifts the spectrum to the right, and results in higher-energy characteristic lines.
- Changing from half-wave to full-wave rectification doubles the height of the spectrum.
- Changing from single-phase to three-phase power results in greater amplitude and a shift to the right on the energy axis.

EXERCISES

1. Which of the following statements applies to the x-ray emission spectrum?
   a. Adding filtration affects characteristic x-ray energy.
   b. Adding filtration affects minimum wavelength.
   c. Adding filtration increases entrance skin exposure.
   d. The target material affects the amplitude of bremsstrahlung x-rays.
   e. The target material affects the minimum wavelength.

2. An increase in mAs results in an increase in:
   a. Average x-ray energy
   b. Both characteristic and bremsstrahlung x-rays
   c. Minimum wavelength
   d. Only the bremsstrahlung x-rays
   e. Only the characteristic x-rays

3. An increase in kVp results in an increase in:
   a. Characteristic x-ray energy
   b. Only the bremsstrahlung x-ray emission spectrum
   c. Only the characteristic x-ray emission spectrum
   d. Radiation quality
   e. Minimum wavelength

4. The intensity of x-ray exposure is best represented by:
   a. The amplitude of the bremsstrahlung x-ray emission spectrum
   b. The amplitude of the characteristic x-ray emission spectrum
   c. The amplitude of the highest emission spectrum
   d. The area under the emission spectrum
   e. The energy range of the emission spectrum

5. Which of the following factors primarily affects the low-energy side of the x-ray emission spectrum?
   a. Exposure time
   b. Filtration
   c. Tube current
   d. Tube voltage
   e. Voltage waveform

6. In general, when changes are made that affect the x-ray emission spectrum and the:
   a. Amplitude increases, the radiation quantity decreases
   b. Line spectrum moves, voltage waveform has changed
   c. Spectrum shifts to the left, a higher-quality beam is emitted
   d. Spectrum shifts to the left, more filtration was used
   e. Spectrum shifts to the right, a more penetrating beam is emitted

Answer the remaining questions about an emission spectrum that represents a diagnostic imaging system operated at 80 kVp/200 mA/100 ms with a tungsten target.

7. How would the bremsstrahlung spectrum change if operation at 80 kVp/200 mA/100 ms were changed to 64 kVp/200 mA/100 ms?
   a. It would remain the same, but the amplitude would decrease.
   b. It would remain the same, but the amplitude would increase.
   c. It would shift to the left and the amplitude would be lower.
   d. It would shift to the left and the amplitude would be higher.
   e. It would shift to the right and the amplitude would be higher.

8. How would the characteristic spectrum change if the operation were at 64 kVp/200 mA/20 ms? The characteristic x-ray spectrum would:
   a. Decrease in height
   b. Disappear
   c. Increase in height
   d. Shift slightly to the left
   e. Shift slightly to the right

Worksheet 9-1
X-Ray Emission
X-Ray Quantity

The intensity of the x-ray beam of an x-ray imaging system is measured in milligray in air and is the **air kerma** (kinetic energy released in **matter**). Radiation exposure **rate** expressed as mGy_a/s, mGy_a/min, or mGy_a/mAs can also be used to express x-ray intensity. Most general-purpose x-ray tubes, when operated at approximately 70 kVp, produce x-ray intensities of approximately 50 $\mu Gy_a/mAs$ at a 100-cm source-to-image receptor distance (SID).

Three adjustable factors affect x-ray quantity:

1. mAs: X-ray quantity is directly proportional to milliampere-seconds (mAs):

$$\frac{I_1}{I_2} = \frac{mAs_1}{mAs_2}$$

2. kVp: X-ray quantity varies approximately as the square of the change in kilovolt peak (kVp):

$$\frac{I_1}{I_2} = (kVp_1/kVp_2)^2$$

3. Distance: X-ray quantity varies inversely with the square of the distance from the target (the inverse square law):

$$I_1/I_2 = (d_2/d_1)^2$$

When these factors are viewed collectively, x-ray exposure of a patient can be estimated at a reasonable approximation with the use of the following equation:

$$\text{x-ray quantity (mR)} = \frac{k(mAs)(kVp)^2}{d^2}$$

where d is the source-to-skin distance (SSD) in centimeters. The constant k will vary from approximately 10 to 30, depending on many factors, including voltage, voltage ripple, filtration, and field size.

EXERCISES

1. When the mAs is increased, the x-ray quantity:
   a. Decreases as the square of the mAs
   b. Decreases proportionately
   c. Increases as the square of the mAs
   d. Increases proportionately
   e. Remains the same

2. When the kVp is increased, the x-ray quantity:
   a. Decreases in proportion to kVp^2
   b. Decreases proportionately
   c. Increases in proportion to kVp^2
   d. Increases proportionately
   e. Remains the same

3. When distance is increased, the x-ray quantity at that distance:
   a. Decreases in proportion to distance squared
   b. Decreases proportionately
   c. Increases in proportion to distance squared
   d. Increases proportionately
   e. Remains the same

4. When x-ray tube filtration is increased, the x-ray quantity:
   a. Decreases
   b. Decreases proportionately
   c. Increases
   d. Increases proportionately
   e. Remains the same

5. In general, x-ray quantity will increase with a/an:
   a. Decrease in exposure time
   b. Decrease in tube current
   c. Increase in distance
   d. Increase in filtration
   e. Increase in kVp

6. X-ray quantity is usually measured as which of the following?
   a. Absorbed dose in mSv
   b. Absorbed dose in Bq
   c. Dose equivalent in Gyt
   d. Exposure in Bq
   e. Exposure in mGya

7. A tungsten-targeted x-ray imaging system is operated at 66 kVp/150 mAs and has an output intensity of 6 mGy_a. Therefore:
   a. Characteristic x-rays will be prominent.
   b. If the mAs is increased to 200, the minimum wavelength will be increased.
   c. Most electron-target atom interactions will result in x-ray emission.
   d. No useful bremsstrahlung radiation will be produced.
   e. The most frequent x-ray emission will be in the 20 to 25 keV range.

8. X-ray quantity can be measured in which of the following?
   a. Bq
   b. Gy_a
   c. Gy_t
   d. Rem
   e. Sv

9. Another meaning of "x-ray quantity" is x-ray:
   a. Energy
   b. Filtration
   c. Intensity
   d. Penetrability
   e. Quality

10. Which of the following does ***not*** affect x-ray quantity?
    a. Filtration
    b. kVp
    c. mA
    d. Radioactivity
    e. Time

11. An extremity radiograph requires 5 mAs and results in an exposure of 180 uGy_a. What will be the exposure if the technique is changed to 7 mAs?
    a. 180 uGy_a
    b. 190 uGy_a
    c. 220 uGy_a
    d. 250 uGy_a
    e. 360 uGy_a

12. An abdominal view is taken at 82 kVp and results in a patient exposure of 1.3 mGy_a. To improve contrast, the kVp is reduced to 74 with no change in mAs. What is the new patient exposure?
    a. 1.1 mGy_a
    b. 1.2 mGy_a
    c. 1.3 mGy_a
    d. 1.5 mGy_a
    e. 1.6 mGy_a

13. A portable chest x-ray is taken at 90 cm SID, and the patient exposure is 280 uGy_a. What will the exposure be if the distance is increased to 180 cm and there is no accompanying technique change?
    a. 70 uGy_a
    b. 120 uGy_a
    c. 170 uGy_a
    d. 630 uGy_a
    e. 1420 uGy_a

14. The output intensity for an x-ray imaging system operated at 70 kVp/400 mA and 50 ms is 0.7 mGy_a. If the mA selector is changed to 600 mA and the exposure time is increased to 80 ms, what will be the output intensity?
    a. 1.05 mGy_a
    b. 1.12 mGy_a
    c. 1.68 mGy_a
    d. 2.10 mGy_a
    e. 2.34 mGy_a

Worksheet 9-2
X-Ray Emission
X-Ray Quality

An x-ray beam that easily penetrates soft tissue and bone is said to be of high quality, whereas a beam that is easily absorbed is of low quality. X-ray quality therefore is a measure of the penetrating ability of an x-ray beam or the energy of the x-ray beam.

- As the voltage of operation is increased, the energy of the x-ray beam is increased; therefore penetrating ability and quality also increase.
- When filtration is added to the beam, it becomes lower quantity, higher energy, and more penetrating, and therefore of greater quality.
- Tube current (mA), exposure time (s), and distance (SID) do not influence the quality of an x-ray beam.
- X-ray beam quality is usually measured by the **half-value layer (HVL)**.
- The HVL is the thickness of an absorber that will reduce the x-ray intensity to one-half of its original value.

EXERCISES

1. Which of the following is the *most* appropriate measure of x-ray beam quality?
   a. Added filtration
   b. HVL
   c. kVp
   d. mAs
   e. Total filtration

2. The quality of an x-ray beam is principally a function of which of the following?
   a. Field size
   b. Filtration
   c. kVp
   d. mAs
   e. SID

3. The HVL is affected principally by a change in which of the following?
   a. Filter thickness
   b. kVp
   c. mAs
   d. SID
   e. X-ray intensity

4. When filtration is added to an x-ray tube, which of the following increases?
   a. Radiation output
   b. Radiation quality
   c. Radiation quantity
   d. SID
   e. SSD

5. Which of the following is the probable HVL of a radiographic x-ray beam at 70 kVp?
   a. 0.5 cm Al
   b. 5.0 cm Al
   c. 0.5 cm soft tissue
   d. 5.0 cm soft tissue
   e. 10 cm soft tissue

6. As filtration is added to an x-ray beam:
   a. All x-rays are removed about equally from the useful beam.
   b. High-energy x-rays are removed more readily than low-energy x-rays.
   c. Low-energy x-rays are removed more readily than high-energy x-rays.
   d. No x-rays are removed, but their average energy is increased.
   e. No x-rays are removed, but their average energy is reduced.

7. An increase in mAs will increase which of the following?
   a. Exposure time
   b. HVL
   c. Total filtration
   d. X-ray quality
   e. X-ray quantity

8. It is often stated that mAs controls quantity and kVp controls:
   a. Collimation
   b. Filtration
   c. Output
   d. Quality
   e. SID

9. However, it should be clear that mAs controls quantity and kVp controls:
   a. Filtration and quality
   b. Output and filtration
   c. Quality and quantity
   d. SID and quality
   e. SID and SSD

10. A minimum HVL is required for diagnostic x-ray beams because:
    a. A greater HVL would mean lower-than-average x-ray energy.
    b. A higher HVL would result in an increased absorbed dose to the patient with no improvement in image quality.
    c. A lower HVL would result in an increased absorbed dose to the patient with no improvement in image quality.
    d. A lower HVL would result in reduced subject contrast.
    e. It protects the operator from excessive scatter.

11. An x-ray beam can be made to have higher effective energy if which of the following occurs?
    a. Filtration is added.
    b. Filtration is removed.
    c. mAs is increased.
    d. SID is increased.
    e. SSD is increased.

12. Which of the following will enhance x-ray beam quality?
    a. Collimation
    b. Filtration
    c. mA
    d. mAs
    e. SID

13. Reducing kVp will do which of the following?
    a. Harden the x-ray beam
    b. Increase the x-ray quality
    c. Increase the x-ray quantity
    d. Require removal of filtration
    e. Soften the x-ray beam

14. Adding filtration to an x-ray beam will do which of the following?
    a. Decrease x-ray quality
    b. Increase inherent filtration
    c. Increase x-ray quality
    d. Increase x-ray quantity
    e. Reduce scatter radiation

15. A radiographic tube has 0.5 mm Al inherent filtration, 1.0 mm Al added filtration, and 1.0 mm Al filtration in the light-localizing collimator. Therefore the total filtration is:
    a. 0.5 mm Al
    b. 1.0 mm Al
    c. 2.0 mm Al
    d. 2.5 mm Al
    e. 4.0 mm Al

Worksheet 9-3 X-Ray Emission Half-Value Layer

Attenuation is the reduction in x-ray beam intensity resulting from photoelectric absorption and Compton scattering of x-rays. The degree of attenuation affects the penetrability of the x-ray beam. Penetrability is one descriptor of the ability of an x-ray beam to pass through tissue and therefore x-ray beam quality. A better descriptor is half-value layer (HVL). The HVL of an x-ray beam is the thickness of absorbing material necessary to reduce the x-ray intensity to half its original value.

The approximate HVL for a diagnostic x-ray beam is:

0.3 mm Pb

3.0 mm Al

3 cm soft tissue

EXERCISES

1. A representative radiographic tube has 0.5 mm Al inherent filtration and 2.0 mm Al added filtration. Therefore:
   a. An additional 1.0 mm Al filtration will harden the x-ray beam.
   b. An additional 1.0 mm Al will increase the x-ray quantity.
   c. An additional 1.0 mm Al will increase total filtration to 3.0 mm Al.
   d. An additional 1.0 mm Al will reduce scatter radiation.
   e. The total filtration is 1.5 mm Al.

2. Which of the following is the softest radiation?
   a. Diagnostic x-rays
   b. Grenz rays
   c. Megavoltage x-rays
   d. Orthovoltage x-rays
   e. Supervoltage x-rays

3. The HVL is defined as:
   a. A thickness of attenuator that will double the x-ray quantity
   b. A thickness of attenuator that will halve the x-ray quantity
   c. Half the required shielding
   d. The mAs value required to double the quantity
   e. Twice the required shielding

4. To measure HVL, which of the following is required?
   a. A collimator
   b. A thermometer
   c. A penetrameter
   d. A spectrometer
   e. Aluminum absorbers

5. As the HVL of a beam increases, its penetrability:
   a. Decreases
   b. Decreases as Z^2
   c. Increases
   d. Increases as Z^2
   e. Is unchanged

6. If increasing the kVp increases the HVL, the x-ray quantity will:
   a. Decrease
   b. Decrease by kVp^2
   c. Increase
   d. Increase by kVp^2
   e. Not change

7. If the HVL is increased by the addition of 1 mm Al, the x-ray quantity will:
   a. Decrease
   b. Decrease by $(mm\ Al)^2$
   c. Increase
   d. Increase by $(mm\ Al)^2$
   e. Not change

8. At 70 kVp, the x-ray beam is attenuated in soft tissue approximately:
   a. 0.05%/cm
   b. 0.5%/cm
   c. 5%/cm
   d. 25%/cm
   e. 50%/cm

9. There is a 75% chance that an x-ray will be attenuated by 2 mm lead. The HVL is:
   a. 0.5 mm Pb
   b. 1.0 mm Pb
   c. 1.5 mm Pb
   d. 2.0 mm Pb
   e. 4.0 mm Pb

10. What occurs when the small rather than the large cathode coil is energized?
    a. Increased cathode heating
    b. Increased x-ray quality
    c. Longer exposures needed
    d. Lower HVL
    e. Smaller effective focal spot

11. Added filtration affects the x-ray beam in what way?
    a. Higher beam quantity
    b. Higher patient dose
    c. Increased beam hardening
    d. Poorer beam quality
    e. Reduced kVp

12. An aluminum filter:
    a. Increases the intensity of all energies of the x-ray beam
    b. Increases skin dose
    c. Is not necessary below 50 kVp
    d. Of at least 1 cm is required
    e. Reduces the effective energy of the beam

13. If patient thickness is 6 HVLs, what is the approximate intensity at the midline of the patient?
    a. 1%
    b. 5%
    c. 12%
    d. 50%
    e. 75%

14. A diagnostic x-ray beam has an HVL of approximately 3 cm soft tissue. What percentage of the beam is absorbed by a 21-cm abdomen?
    a. 0 to 10
    b. 10 to 20
    c. 20 to 60
    d. 60 to 90
    e. >90

15. Which is reduced as x-ray energy increases?
    a. Filtration
    b. Projectile-electron energy
    c. Target-electron energy
    d. X-ray frequency
    e. X-ray wavelength

16. An increase in kVp results in an increase in:
    a. Characteristic x-ray energy
    b. Only the bremsstrahlung x-ray emission spectrum
    c. Only the characteristic x-ray emission spectrum
    d. Radiation quality
    e. The maximum x-ray wavelength

17. An x-ray beam HVL can be increased by increasing which of the following?
    a. Filtration
    b. mA
    c. mAs
    d. SID
    e. SSD

18. The HVL is affected most by a change in:
    a. Added filtration
    b. kVp
    c. mAs
    d. SID
    e. X-ray intensity

19. The added filtration in a conventional light-localizing variable aperture collimator is:
    a. 0 mm Al
    b. 0.5 mm Al
    c. 1.0 mm Al
    d. 3.0 mm Al
    e. 10 mm Al

Worksheet 9-4 X-Ray Emission Filtration

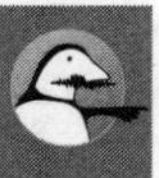

Three types of x-ray beam filtration exist:

- **Inherent filtration**: This results from the glass or metal envelope of the x-ray tube and the window in the x-ray tube housing. It is usually equivalent to approximately 0.5 mm Al.
- **Added filtration**: This is the result of placing an absorber in the path of the x-ray beam. The absorber, usually 1 to 3 mm Al, is positioned between the collimator and the tube housing.
- **Compensating filtration**: This has nothing to do with patient dose; compensating filters are used specifically for shaping the x-ray intensity over the beam area so that radiation that reaches the image receptor is more uniform and produces more uniform optical density.

EXERCISES

1. The inherent filtration in a general-purpose radiographic x-ray tube is usually equivalent to:
   a. 0 mm Al
   b. 0.1 mm Al
   c. 0.5 mm Al
   d. 1.0 mm Al
   e. 2.5 mm Al

2. The equivalent added filtration provided by a conventional light-localizing, variable-aperture collimator is closest to:
   a. 0 mm Al
   b. 0.5 mm Al
   c. 1.0 mm Al
   d. 2.0 mm Al
   e. 2.5 mm Al

3. The purpose of a wedge filter in diagnostic radiology is to produce:
   a. A harder beam
   b. A softer beam
   c. A uniform x-ray beam intensity at the image receptor
   d. A uniform x-ray beam intensity at the patient
   e. An x-ray beam to fit the image receptor

4. The primary purpose of adding filtration to an x-ray beam is to:
   a. Cause high-energy x-rays to Compton scatter
   b. Protect the image receptor from low-energy x-rays
   c. Remove low-energy electrons
   d. Remove low-energy x-rays
   e. Remove penetrating x-rays

5. An x-ray beam filter has the *greatest* effect on dose reduction to the:
   a. Gonads
   b. Lens
   c. Skin
   d. Thyroid
   e. Whole body

6. X-rays of higher maximum energy can be obtained by doing which of the following?
   a. Increasing filtration
   b. Increasing kVp
   c. Increasing mAs
   d. Reducing inherent filtration
   e. Using a higher Z target

7. The light-localizing, variable-aperture collimator contributes:
   a. No filtration when its light is off
   b. No filtration when its light is on
   c. Scatter x-rays
   d. To added filtration
   e. To inherent filtration

8. If 5-mm Al filtration is added to the x-ray tube:
   a. Contrast resolution will improve.
   b. Motion unsharpness will decrease.
   c. Beam energy will increase.
   d. Patient dose will increase.
   e. Radiographic contrast will increase.

9. An x-ray beam can be made harder by increasing which of the following?
   a. Filtration
   b. mA
   c. mAs
   d. SID
   e. SSD

10. When filtration is added to a normally filtered x-ray beam, the x-ray emission spectrum will:
   a. Decrease in amplitude
   b. Have higher-energy discrete lines
   c. Have lower-energy discrete lines
   d. Increase in amplitude
   e. Shift to the left

11. Added filtration:
   a. Increases x-ray quantity
   b. Is expensive
   c. Is usually thinner than inherent filtration
   d. Protects the patient from unnecessary radiation exposure
   e. Reduces x-ray quality

12. Inherent filtration:
   a. Consists of sheets of aluminum
   b. Helps harden the x-ray beam
   c. Is approximately 2.0 mm Al
   d. Is mainly due to the light localizer
   e. Tends to decrease with tube age

13. To produce low inherent filtration in an x-ray beam:
   a. A thin section of glass is used.
   b. Insulating oil is placed around the tube.
   c. kVp should be reduced.
   d. The collimator should be removed.
   e. Windows made of copper are used.

14. Wedge filters are:
   a. Always better than uniform filters because they attenuate a greater number of x-rays
   b. Used for lateral skull examinations
   c. Used to image a knee
   d. Used to match the image receptor
   e. Used to obtain uniform optical density

15. When added filtration is increased:
   a. kVp must be reduced.
   b. mAs must be reduced.
   c. Effective x-ray energy is reduced.
   d. X-ray quality is enhanced.
   e. X-ray quantity is increased.

16. If a radiographic tube has 0.5 mm Al inherent filtration and 2.0 mm Al added filtration, which of the following is *true?*
   a. Adding 1.0 mm Al will harden the x-ray beam.
   b. Adding 1.0 mm Al will increase the total filtration to 2.5 mm Al.
   c. Adding 1.0 mm Al will increase the x-ray quantity.
   d. Removing 1.0 mm Al will increase HVL.
   e. The total filtration is 1.5 mm Al.

17. Inherent filtration is:
   a. Dependent on the type of aluminum used
   b. Increased when kVp is raised
   c. Increased with patient thickness
   d. Increased with tube age
   e. Produced by slowing down electrons

18. An x-ray tube has a total filtration of 3.0 mm Al, an HVL of 2.5 mm Al, and emits 1.8 mGy_a. Therefore:
   a. The addition of 1.0 mm Al filtration will increase the quantity of the beam.
   b. The addition of 1.0 mm Al will enhance the quality of the beam.
   c. The addition of 2.5 mm Al will reduce the output intensity to 1 mGy_a.
   d. The addition of 2.5 mm Al will reduce the output intensity to 1.35 mGy_a.
   e. The output is also 0.07 mGy_a/mAs.

Worksheet 10-1
X-Ray Interaction With Matter
Compton Effect

X-ray interaction with loosely bound electrons of tissue atoms is responsible for scatter radiation. The incident x-ray interacts with an outer-shell electron of a tissue atom and transfers some of its energy to the electron. After the interaction, the electron is ejected from the atom (the atom is ionized) and the x-ray is scattered. Because the incident x-ray imparts some of its energy to the Compton electron, it loses energy.

The probability that an x-ray will undergo a Compton interaction decreases with increasing x-ray energy. The occurrence of the Compton effect is independent of the atomic number of the absorber. In conventional radiography, more than 70% of the incident x-rays undergo Compton interactions; this interaction contributes to the radiographic noise that reduces contrast.

EXERCISES

1. Which of the following is ***not*** one of the five basic x-ray interactions with matter?
   a. Bremsstrahlung
   b. Classical scattering
   c. Compton scattering
   d. Photodisintegration
   e. Photoelectric effect

2. Which of the following x-rays would be ***most*** likely to undergo classical scattering?
   a. 5 keV
   b. 15 keV
   c. 35 keV
   d. 66 keV
   e. 85 keV

3. Which of the following interactions contributes to image noise?
   a. Bremsstrahlung
   b. Characteristic
   c. Compton scattering
   d. Photodisintegration
   e. Photoelectric effect

4. Which of the following occurs in a Compton interaction?
   a. An atom is excited.
   b. An atom is ionized.
   c. The secondary electron has kinetic energy equal to the difference between the energy of the incident x-ray and the electron-binding energy.
   d. The secondary electron has kinetic energy equal to the incident x-ray.
   e. The secondary photon has a wavelength equal to the primary x-ray.

5. If E_i = incident x-ray energy, E_s = scattered x-ray energy, E_b = electron-binding energy, and E_{KE} = secondary electron kinetic energy, then which of the following is *true?*
   a. $E_i = E_s + E_b + E_{KE}$
   b. $E_i = E_s - E_b - E_{KE}$
   c. $E_i = E_s - E_b + E_{KE}$
   d. $E_i = E_s + (E_b - E_{KE})$
   e. $E_i = E_{KE} - (E_b + E_s)$

6. If E_i = incident x-ray energy, E_s = scattered x-ray energy, E_b = electron-binding energy, and E_{KE} = secondary electron kinetic energy, then which of the following is *true?*
   a. $E_s = E_b + E_{KE} + E_i$
   b. $E_s = E_b - (E_{KE} + E_i)$
   c. $E_s = E_{KE} - (E_b + E_i)$
   d. $E_s = E_i - (E_b + E_{KE})$
   e. $E_s = E_{KE} + E_i - E_b$

7. During the Compton effect, *most* of the incident x-ray energy is given to which of the following?
   a. Characteristic radiation
   b. Excitation
   c. Electron-binding energy
   d. Electron mass
   e. Scattered x-ray

8. After Compton scattering, the scattered x-ray has:
   a. Higher energy
   b. Higher frequency
   c. Less mass
   d. Longer wavelength
   e. Lower velocity

9. Compton interaction affects the image by increasing which of the following?
   a. Contrast resolution
   b. Latitude
   c. Fog
   d. Spatial resolution
   e. Grid Ratio

10. The probability that an x-ray will interact with an outer-shell electron is influenced principally by:
    a. The atomic number of the absorber
    b. The binding energy of the electron
    c. The energy of the incident x-ray
    d. The kinetic energy of the electron
    e. The x-ray production mode

11. The Compton effect is:
    a. Independent of Z
    b. Inversely proportional to Z
    c. Proportional to E
    d. Proportional to Z
    e. Proportional to Z^2

12. The Compton effect is:
    a. Also called classical scattering
    b. The principal source of image noise (fog)
    c. The same as Rayleigh scattering
    d. The same as the Thomson effect
    e. The source of the latent image

13. If a 45 keV x-ray interacts with the K-shell electron in an atom of molybdenum ($E_b = 20$ keV) and ejects it with 8 keV energy, what will be the energy of the scattered x-ray?
    a. 12 keV
    b. 17 keV
    c. 25 keV
    d. 37 keV
    e. 45 keV

14. The probability that an x-ray will undergo Compton interaction:
    a. Decreases with increasing x-ray energy
    b. Increases with decreasing electron energy
    c. Increases with increasing electron energy
    d. Increases with increasing x-ray energy
    e. Increases with increasing Z of the target atom

15. The Compton interaction involves so-called "unbound" electrons because:
    a. Excitation occurs.
    b. Free electrons are ejected.
    c. Ionization occurs.
    d. K-shell electrons are not involved.
    e. They have a very low binding energy.

16. Which of the following is the x-ray interaction that does *not* cause ionization?
    a. Classical scattering
    b. Compton scattering
    c. Pair production
    d. Photodisintegration
    e. Photoelectric effect

17. Compton-scattered x-rays:
    a. Are helpful in diagnostic radiology
    b. Have lower energy than the incident x-ray
    c. Improve contrast resolution
    d. Produce image artifacts
    e. Result from bremsstrahlung

Worksheet 10-2
X-Ray Interaction With Matter
Photoelectric Effect

The photoelectric effect occurs when an incident x-ray imparts all its energy to an orbital electron of a tissue atom, usually a K-shell electron. The x-ray disappears, and the orbital electron is ejected from the atom. This electron is a **photoelectron**, and it escapes with kinetic energy equal to the difference between the incident x-ray energy and its binding energy.

The probability that a given x-ray will undergo a photoelectric interaction is **inversely** proportional to the third power of the photon energy ($1/E^3$) and **directly** proportional to the third power of the atomic number (Z^3) of the absorber.

Photoelectric effect results in image contrast. Contrast agent studies incorporating barium or iodine are successful because the atomic number of these atoms is much higher than that of the atoms of surrounding tissue.

EXERCISES

1. If E_i = incident x-ray energy, E_s = scattered x-ray energy, E_b = electron-binding energy, and E_{KE} = photoelectric kinetic energy, then which of the following is *true?*
   a. $E_i = E_s + E_b + E_{KE}$
   b. $E_i = E_s - (E_b + E_{KE})$
   c. $E_i = E_b + E_{KE}$
   d. $E_i = E_b - E_{KE}$
   e. $E_i = E_{KE} - E_b$

2. If E_i = incident x-ray energy, E_s = scattered x-ray energy, E_b = electron-binding energy, and E_{KE} = photoelectric kinetic energy, then which of the following is *true?*
   a. $E_{KE} = E_i - E_b$
   b. $E_{KE} = E_i/E_b$
   c. $E_s = E_i - (E_b + E_{KE})$
   d. $E_s = (E_b + E_{KE})\ E_i$
   e. $E_i = E_s + E_b + E_{KE}$

3. The photoelectric effect is principally associated with which of the following?
   a. Absorption of an x-ray
   b. Bremsstrahlung x-ray production
   c. Characteristic x-ray production
   d. Electron excitation
   e. Scattering of an x-ray

4. A 50 keV x-ray has a 0.02 chance of photoelectric interaction with muscle (Z = 7.4). What is its chance of interacting with bone (Z = 13.8)?
   a. 0.01
   b. 0.04
   c. 0.07
   d. 0.14
   e. 0.37

5. Which of the following has the lowest effective atomic number?
   a. Air
   b. Bone
   c. Fat
   d. Lung
   e. Muscle

6. Photoelectric interaction with soft tissue is *most* likely with which of the following x-rays?
   a. 0.3 keV
   b. 3.0 keV
   c. 30 keV
   d. 300 keV
   e. 3000 keV

7. During photoelectric interaction:
   a. An electron is emitted from the atom.
   b. An x-ray is emitted from the atom.
   c. Electron excitation results.
   d. The atom is made radioactive.
   e. The incident x-ray reappears with reduced energy.

8. During operation at 80 kVp, which of the following photoelectric interactions is most probable?
   a. 30 keV x-ray and bone
   b. 30 keV x-ray and fat
   c. 50 keV x-ray and lung
   d. 70 keV x-ray and bone
   e. 70 keV x-ray and fat

9. The radiographic image is formed principally by which of the following?
   a. Classical scattering
   b. Compton scattering
   c. Off-focus radiation
   d. Photoelectric interactions
   e. Uniform distribution of remnant x-rays

10. A 35 keV x-ray ***most*** likely will undergo K-shell photoelectric interaction with which of the following?
    a. Barium ($E_b = 37$ keV)
    b. Calcium ($E_b = 4$ keV)
    c. Iodine ($E_b = 33$ keV)
    d. Muscle ($E_b < 1$ keV)
    e. Tungsten ($E_b = 69$ keV)

11. The probability of photoelectric effect varies as what function of x-ray energy (E)?
    a. E^{-3}
    b. E^{-2}
    c. E
    d. E^2
    e. E^3

12. As a result of photoelectric interaction:
    a. An electron is absorbed.
    b. An electron leaves the atom.
    c. The incident x-ray is scattered.
    d. The incident x-ray leaves the atom with more energy.
    e. The incident x-ray leaves the atom with reduced energy.

13. The photoelectric effect is:
    a. A partially exciting event
    b. A partially ionizing event
    c. A radiation-scattering event
    d. The complete absorption of an electron with the subsequent emission of an x-ray
    e. The complete absorption of an x-ray with the subsequent emission of an electron

14. Lead has a K-shell electron-binding energy of 88 keV. Therefore:
    a. An 84 keV x-ray can undergo photoelectric interaction with the K-shell electron.
    b. An 84 keV x-ray can undergo photoelectric interaction with the L-shell electron.
    c. An 87 keV x-ray is more likely to undergo photoelectric interaction with a K-shell electron than an 84 keV x-ray.
    d. An 87 keV x-ray is more likely to undergo photoelectric interaction with an L-shell electron than an 84 keV x-ray.
    e. An 87 keV x-ray will be replaced by a 1 keV electron.

15. A 39 keV x-ray interacts through a photoelectric effect with a K-shell electron of barium (binding energy 37 keV). Therefore:
    a. The photoelectron will have 2 keV energy.
    b. The photoelectron will have 37 keV energy.
    c. The photoelectron will have 39 keV energy.
    d. The scattered x-ray will have 2 keV energy.
    e. The scattered x-ray will have 37 keV energy.

16. The probability of photoelectric effect varies as what function of target atomic number (Z)?
    a. Z^{-3}
    b. Z^{-2}
    c. Z
    d. Z^2
    e. Z^3

Worksheet 10-3 X-Ray Interaction With Matter Differential Absorption/Atomic Number

- Only two interactions of the incident x-ray are important to diagnostic x-ray imaging: Compton scattering and the photoelectric effect. The photoelectric effect predominates when low-energy x-rays interact with atoms that have a high atomic number.
- Compton scattering predominates at high voltage, where it accounts for most of the interactions between x-rays and tissue.
- Both interactions are equally proportional to mass density.
- However, the ratio of Compton scattering to the photoelectric effect increases with increasing x-ray energy.
- The pattern of absorption and scatter of the incident x-ray beam caused by atomic number, mass density, and thickness of tissue is called **differential absorption**.

EXERCISES

1. Anatomic structures that readily transmit x-rays:
   a. Are called *radiolucent*
   b. Are called *radiopaque*
   c. Have a high effective atomic number
   d. Have a high probability for photoelectric effect
   e. Usually have high mass density

2. Differential absorption, although a complicated process, is basically the result of differences between:
   a. Compton scattering and photoelectric effect
   b. Compton scattering and transmission
   c. High-E and low-E x-rays
   d. High-Z and low-Z tissue
   e. Photoelectric effect and transmission

3. When a radiograph is taken:
   a. High kVp is preferred for maximum differential absorption.
   b. Low kVp is necessary when soft tissue is imaged because it leads to high Compton effect.
   c. Low kVp is necessary when soft tissue is imaged because it leads to high photoelectric effect.
   d. The most probable interaction is no interaction.
   e. With increasing kVp, differential absorption increases.

4. At what approximate x-ray energy is the probability of a photoelectric interaction in soft tissue equal to the probability of a Compton interaction?
   a. 10 keV
   b. 20 keV
   c. 40 keV
   d. 80 keV
   e. 120 keV

5. Which of the following has the greatest mass density?
   a. Blood
   b. Bone
   c. Fat
   d. Lung
   e. Muscle

6. The colon is imaged during a barium enema examination principally because of differences in:
   a. Beam energy
   b. Beam intensity
   c. Subject atomic number
   d. Subject mass density
   e. Subject mass number

7. Air-contrast studies such as a colon examination are successful principally for which of the following reasons?
   a. High-kVp technique is used.
   b. Low-kVp technique is used.
   c. There are differences in effective x-ray energy.
   d. There are differences in mass density.
   e. X-rays are produced with a continuous-energy spectrum.

8. To optimize x-ray mammography:
   a. High kVp is required to minimize Compton effect.
   b. High kVp should be used with adequate filtration.
   c. Low kVp is necessary to take advantage of Compton effect.
   d. Low kVp is required because of high Z of microcalcifications.
   e. The main x-ray interaction should be the photoelectric effect.

9. Differential absorption between bone and soft tissue occurs principally for which of the following reasons?
   a. There is a difference in effective atomic number.
   b. There is a difference in mass density.
   c. There is a difference in reflectance.
   d. The x-ray beam is monoenergetic.
   e. The x-ray beam is polyenergetic.

10. Angiography with iodinated compounds:
    a. Requires high kVp for high contrast
    b. Works because of the Compton effect
    c. Works principally because of differences in effective atomic number
    d. Works principally because of differences in mass density
    e. Would not be possible with monoenergetic x-rays

11. Differential absorption is:
    a. Better with increasing Compton interaction
    b. Better with increasing kVp
    c. Better with thicker anatomy
    d. The difference between those x-rays that are absorbed and those that are reflected
    e. The difference between those x-rays that are absorbed and those that are transmitted

12. As kVp increases, the relative number of x-rays:
    a. That is reflected decreases
    b. That is transmitted decreases
    c. That interacts by way of the Compton effect increases
    d. That interacts by way of the photoelectric effect increases
    e. That interacts with tissue decreases

13. In which of the following tissues does differential absorption *most* depend on differences in mass density?
    a. Fat and bone
    b. Lung and bone
    c. Lung and fat
    d. Muscle and bone
    e. Muscle and fat

14. The SI unit of mass density is which of the following?
    a. m^3/g
    b. g/m^3
    c. kg/m^3
    d. Joule
    e. Newton

15. How is photoelectric interaction with tissue related to the mass density (ρ) of the tissue?
    a. It is inversely proportional.
    b. It is inversely proportional to ρ^3.
    c. It is proportional.
    d. It is proportional to ρ^3.
    e. It is unrelated.

16. Lungs are imaged on a chest radiograph principally because of differences in which of the following?
    a. Beam energy
    b. Beam intensity
    c. Tissue atomic number
    d. Tissue mass density
    e. Tissue mass number

Worksheet 10-4
X-Ray Interaction With Matter
Differential Absorption/Mass Density

Differential absorption occurs because of differences in photoelectric absorption and Compton scattering, both of which attenuate the x-ray beam. Image-forming x-rays consist of those transmitted through the patient and the Compton scattered x-rays.

Differential absorption is less with increasing x-ray beam energy. However, the interaction of x-rays with tissue is proportional to the mass density of the tissue regardless of x-ray quantity, quality, or the type of interaction.

EXERCISES

1. Differential absorption between lung and soft tissue occurs principally because of which of the following?
   a. The difference in effective atomic numbers (Z)
   b. The difference in mass density
   c. The x-ray beam is filtered.
   d. The x-ray beam is homogeneous.
   e. The x-ray beam is polyenergetic.

2. The reduction in intensity of an x-ray beam after it passes through tissue is called:
   a. Absorption
   b. Attenuation
   c. Exponential
   d. Interaction
   e. Scattering

3. X-ray transmission decreases exponentially, which also means that:
   a. Beam intensity is reduced abruptly.
   b. The number of x-rays is never reduced to zero.
   c. The x-ray beam becomes more penetrating.
   d. There is a finite thickness for 100% absorption.
   e. X-ray scattering increases.

4. Which process contributes *most* to the radiographic image?
   a. Classical scattering
   b. Compton scattering
   c. Pair production
   d. Photodisintegration
   e. Photoelectric effect

5. High kVp in chest radiography will:
   a. Increase contrast
   b. Increase patient dose
   c. Increase noise
   d. Reduce patient dose
   e. Reduce shadowing from the rib

6. Increasing kVp in x-ray imaging will:
   a. Increase contrast
   b. Increase filtration
   c. Decrease magnification
   d. Reduce source-to-image receptor distance (SID)
   e. Reduce skin dose

7. In high-kVp chest radiography, contrast depends *most* on:
   a. Atomic number
   b. mAs
   c. Mass density
   d. Mass number
   e. SID

8. Microcalcifications are imaged on mammograms principally because of:
   a. Atomic number
   b. Atomic mass
   c. Electron density
   d. Mass density
   e. SID

9. More contrast is present from a barium examination than from an iodine examination because:
   a. Barium has a higher atomic number.
   b. Barium has a higher concentration.
   c. Barium has a higher mass attenuation coefficient.
   d. Iodine has a higher atomic number.
   e. The luminal size is greater for the colon than for the ureter.

10. Photoelectric effect is proportional to:
    a. $E^{-1/2}$
    b. $E^{1/2}$
    c. E^3
    d. $Z^{1/2}$
    e. Z^3

11. What will increase the energy of bremsstrahlung radiation?
    a. Filament current
    b. Exposure time
    c. SID
    d. Target material
    e. X-ray tube voltage

12. Compton interaction occurs with outer-shell electrons and results in:
    a. Auger electron + photon of lower energy
    b. Conversion electron + photon of lower energy
    c. Electron capture + characteristic x-ray
    d. Recoil electron + photon of higher energy
    e. Reduced grayscale

13. At 60 keV in soft tissue, what predominates?
    a. Classical scattering
    b. Compton scattering
    c. Pair production
    d. Photodisintegration
    e. Photoelectric effect

14. Compton interaction affects the image by increasing which of the following?
    a. Contrast resolution
    b. Latitude
    c. Fog
    d. Spatial resolution
    e. Magnification

15. Differential absorption in which of the following tissues is most dependent on differences in mass density?
    a. Fat and bone
    b. Lung and bone
    c. Lung and fat
    d. Muscle and bone
    e. Muscle and fat

16. Fat has a higher concentration of hydrogen than soft tissue; therefore which of the following is higher in fat than in soft tissue?
    a. Mass density
    b. Effective atomic number
    c. Electron density
    d. X-ray absorption above 100 keV
    e. X-ray absorption below 30 keV

17. Differential absorption:
    a. Increases with increasing Compton scatter
    b. Increases with increasing kVp
    c. Is the difference between absorbed x-rays and reflected x-rays
    d. Is the difference between absorbed x-rays and transmitted x-rays
    e. Is improved with higher mAs

Worksheet 11-1
Computed Radiography Image Receptor

Computed radiography (CR) first appeared in 1984, but it took a decade for CR to become clinically acceptable. CR was the first example of digital radiography. Wet chemistry processing of a latent image is replaced with laser stimulation of metastable electrons that serve as the latent image.

The image receptor in CR is a photostimulable phosphor (PSP) made of barium fluorohalide such as barium fluorobromide (BaFlBr). It appears physically much like a radiographic intensifying screen. With a PSP, however, no light is emitted in response to x-ray exposure. Rather, electrons are energized into a metastable state by the interaction of x-rays.

When an intense laser light is incident on the PSP, light is emitted as the metastable electrons return to their ground state. The intensity of this laser-stimulated light is proportional to the x-ray intensity at the image receptor.

EXERCISES

1. The laser light used in CR:
   a. Is in the ultraviolet light region
   b. Is more energetic than the stimulated light
   c. Is pulsed across the PSP
   d. Has a longer wavelength than the stimulated light
   e. Produces light of intense fluorescence

2. An electron that is being described as metastable:
   a. Is outside the atom
   b. Is present in positive and negative forms
   c. Is the transformation of an x-ray
   d. Has been captured by the nucleus
   e. Has higher energy than it should have

3. Doping of a PSP with europium results in:
   a. Better contrast resolution
   b. Better spatial resolution
   c. Higher x-ray absorption
   d. Lower patient dose
   e. More stimulable light emission

4. The activator in a PSP is there to:
   a. Define laser wavelength
   b. Enhance electron metastability
   c. Increase x-ray absorption
   d. Select the proper wavelength
   e. Shape the wavelength of stimulable emission

5. Which of the following is most intense?
   a. Laser light
   b. Normal visual light
   c. Optical lens support
   d. Stimulable emission
   e. X-ray beam

6. Which of the following is monochromatic?
   a. Infrared light
   b. Laser light
   c. Stimulated emission
   d. Visible light
   e. X-ray beam

7. PSP image receptors are effective because:
   a. Metastable states are produced.
   b. Contrast is proportional to dose.
   c. Spatial resolution is improved.
   d. Their response follows the H & D curve.
   e. They are composed of detector elements.

8. About how much time can pass between exposing a CR plate and reading a CR plate before image quality declines?
   a. 1 hour
   b. 10 minutes
   c. 8 hours
   d. 3 weeks
   e. 6 days

9. As a descriptor of a PSP, the term *turbid* refers to an appearance that is:
   a. Black
   b. Clear
   c. Colored
   d. Cloudy
   e. Gray

10. Europium is an activator in the PSP. An activator is responsible for:
    a. Contrast resolution
    b. Emitted light intensity
    c. Reduced patient dose
    d. Spatial resolution
    e. X-ray absorption

11. PSP image receptors:
    a. Are relatively insensitive to x-rays
    b. Become radiation fatigued with age
    c. Can be fogged by background radiation
    d. Do not require processing
    e. Require higher patient dose

12. To remove the image of background radiation or a previous image, one should:
    a. Clear the image receptor with a cleaning solution.
    b. Expose the image receptor to intense light.
    c. Expose the image receptor to intense x-ray exposure.
    d. Store the image receptor for 3 days.
    e. Transfer the image receptor signal to digital storage.

13. Which of the following is the proper sequence for producing a computed radiographic image?
    a. Erase/read/expose
    b. Expose/erase/read
    c. Expose/read/erase
    d. Read/erase/expose
    e. Read/expose/erase

14. Thermoluminescent dosimeters emit light when:
    a. Exposed to heat
    b. Exposed to light
    c. Exposed to x-rays
    d. Exposed to cold
    e. Exposed to gamma rays

15. PSP emit light when:
    a. Exposed to heat
    b. Exposed to light
    c. Exposed to x-rays
    d. Exposed to cold
    e. Exposed to gamma rays

16. Fog will appear on the CR plate with exposure to:
    a. Light
    b. Background radiation
    c. Laser light
    d. Humidity
    e. Cold

17. CR plates eliminate the need for:
    a. A processor
    b. Proper patient positioning
    c. Techniques that minimize dose
    d. A darkroom
    e. Computers

Worksheet 11-2 Computed Radiography Reader

Inside the computed radiography reader are mechanical drive mechanisms, optical shaping lenses and mirrors, and photosensitive detectors. The mechanical drive mechanism supports a "slow" scan of the imaging plate by moving the plate slowly through the reader. The optical assembly supports a "fast" scan mode by deflecting the laser beam back and forth across the imaging plate as it is slowly scanned.

Interaction of the laser beam with the imaging plate results in photostimulable emission, which is measured by a photodiode and quantified. The intensity of photostimulable emission is proportional to the intensity of the x-ray exposure to that portion of the imaging plate. The diameter of the laser beam and scan motion determine the size of each pixel.

EXERCISES

1. The photostimulable emission in computed radiography (CR):
   a. Has longer wavelength than the laser-stimulating light
   b. Has shorter wavelength than the laser-stimulating light
   c. Is discrete, as is the laser-stimulating light
   d. Is in the far infrared region of the spectrum
   e. Is monochromatic, as is the laser-stimulating light

2. The slow-scan portion of the CR reader:
   a. Has a speed that is determined by the emission rate
   b. Is under mechanical control
   c. Is under optical control
   d. Relies on a photometric response
   e. Requires mirrors and prisms

3. Spatial resolution in CR is principally determined by:
   a. Fast-scan rate
   b. Field of view
   c. Laser beam diameter
   d. Phosphor size
   e. Slow-scan rate

4. The source of the stimulating light is:
   a. Emitted light
   b. The laser
   c. The optical path
   d. The photometer
   e. X-radiation

5. What is the approximate diameter of the laser beam?
   a. <1 nm
   b. 10 nm
   c. 100 nm
   d. 1000 nm
   e. >1000 nm

6. How does the CR reader maintain the laser beam as a circle?
   a. Beam-shaping optics
   b. Fast-scan regulation
   c. Intensity control
   d. Light-collecting optics
   e. Slow-scan regulation

7. Which of the following is *not* a photodetector?
   a. ADC
   b. CCD
   c. CMOS
   d. PD
   e. PMT

8. The x-ray capture element of a CR imaging plate is the:
   a. BaFlBr
   b. Cassette
   c. CCD
   d. Laser beam
   e. Light-collecting optics

9. The characteristic curve of a CR imaging plate is described as:
   a. Detective quantum efficiency
   b. Image buffer
   c. Image receptor response function
   d. Modulation transfer function
   e. Sampling quantization

10. Patient radiation dose reduction in computed radiography is limited by:
    a. Fast-scan mode
    b. Image contrast
    c. Patient size
    d. Slow-scan mode
    e. System noise

11. A CR image receptor is responsive to an x-ray beam over how many orders of magnitude?
    a. One
    b. Two
    c. Three
    d. Four
    e. Five

12. Which of the following is a source of image noise that is apparent in CR?
    a. Latent image fading
    b. Electronic noise
    c. Noise due to properties of the phosphor
    d. Image receptor noise
    e. Scatter

13. CR imaging allows for the display of about:
    a. 30 shades of gray
    b. 100 shades of gray
    c. 3000 shades of gray
    d. 10,000 shades of gray
    e. 1 billion shades of gray

Worksheet 12-1
Direct Radiography

Direct radiography produces digital radiographic images with a flat-panel, solid-state image receptor. Three designs are in use: photostimulable phosphor charge-coupled device (CCD), amorphous silicon (a-Si), and amorphous selenium (a-Se).

EXERCISES

1. Which of the following is the principal disadvantage of using an area beam versus scanned projection radiography (SPR)?
   a. Increased patient dose
   b. Lack of postexamination processing
   c. Reduced spatial resolution
   d. Scatter radiation
   e. Short exposure time

2. In scanned projection digital radiography, which of the following moves to produce an image?
   a. The x-ray tube
   b. A CCD
   c. A laser
   d. The patient
   e. The image receptor

3. An SPR:
   a. Has better spatial resolution
   b. Has worse contrast than digital fluoroscopy
   c. Is like a tomograph
   d. Is virtually scatter-free
   e. Removes superposition of structures

4. Which of the following is a part of SPR?
   a. Analog-to-digital converter
   b. Area beam
   c. Data acquisition system
   d. Detector array
   e. Video monitor

5. The principal advantage of using an area beam versus SPR is which of the following?
   a. Improved contrast resolution
   b. Low patient dose
   c. Postexamination processing
   d. Scatter radiation rejection
   e. Short exposure time

6. Which of the following is an advantage of an area beam over SPR in digital radiography?
   a. Improved contrast
   b. Less scatter
   c. Less technique required
   d. Low noise
   e. Reduced motion blur

7. Which of the following is used as an image receptor in direct radiography?
   a. An image intensifier
   b. $CaWO_4$
   c. $CdWO_4$
   d. a-Se
   e. Rare earth phosphors

8. The principal disadvantage of digital radiography is?
   a. Edge enhancement
   b. Longer exposure time
   c. More motion artifact
   d. Poor contrast resolution
   e. Poor spatial resolution

9. A digital image constructed on a 512×512 matrix will have how many pixels?
   a. 512
   b. 1024
   c. 512^2
   d. 1024^2
   e. 1636

10. All of the following are materials used in direct radiography except:
    a. a-Se
    b. CsI
    c. GdOS
    d. CCD
    e. LaOBr

11. Which of the following is unique to direct radiography?
    a. A detector array
    b. Area x-ray beam
    c. Fast image access
    d. No scintillation phosphor
    e. Reregistration

12. The image receptor in computed radiography could be:
    a. a-Se
    b. a-Si
    c. BaFlCl
    d. $CaWO_4$
    e. $CdWO_4$

13. Which of the following is used as a radiation detector in direct radiography?
    a. BGO
    b. $CdWO_4$
    c. Ceramic
    d. a-Se
    e. Xe

14. The principal limitation of the SPR mode of digital radiography is which of the following?
    a. Cost
    b. Examination time
    c. Image noise
    d. Patient dose
    e. Spatial resolution

15. An x-ray system used for direct radiography has which of the following?
    a. A linear characteristic curve
    b. Photostimulable phosphor (PSP)
    c. A rapid charger
    d. Access to the Internet
    e. At least two video monitors

16. Spatial resolution in digital imaging systems is primarily limited by:
    a. Speed of the examination
    b. The amount of collimation
    c. The tube's heat capacity
    d. Scatter
    e. Size and number of detectors

17. The principal advantage of a fan-shaped x-ray beam over an area x-ray beam is which of the following?
    a. Examination time
    b. Hybrid images
    c. Less heat generated
    d. Reduced patient dose
    e. Scatter radiation rejection

18. Which of the following has the highest spatial resolution?
    a. Computed radiography
    b. Direct radiography
    c. SPR
    d. Digital mammography
    e. Computed tomography

19. Which is most important for soft tissue contrast?
    a. Contrast resolution
    b. Spatial resolution
    c. High lp/mm
    d. Noise
    e. Scatter

Worksheet 13-1 Spatial Resolution

The ability of an imaging system to render on the image a faithful reproduction of a small, high-contrast object is termed **spatial resolution**. The smaller the object that can be imaged, the better the spatial resolution.

It is easy to image smaller and smaller objects and to state spatial resolution in terms of object size—1 cm, 1 mm, or 1 μm. In medical imaging, spatial resolution is expressed in terms of spatial frequency—frequency in space. Spatial frequency is a measure of how quickly an object changes in space.

Tissues can be identified by their spatial frequency. Calcified lung nodules or breast microcalcifications are high spatial frequency objects. Abdominal tissue, fat, and soft tissue masses are low spatial frequency objects. It is difficult for any imaging system to image both high-frequency and low-frequency objects.

As a generalization, digital imaging systems have better contrast resolution but poorer spatial resolution than previous imaging systems.

EXERCISES

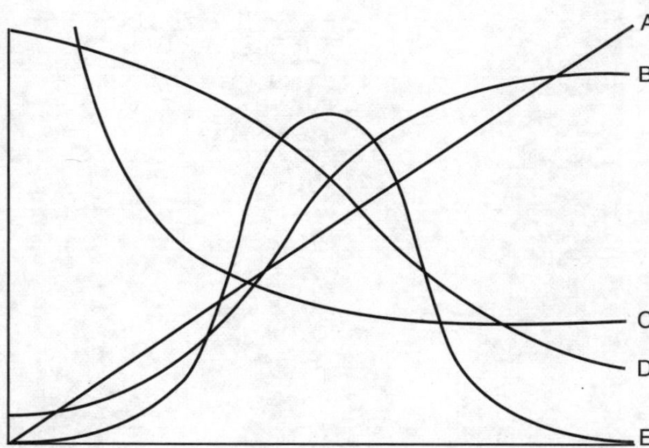

Use the figure above to answer Questions 1 through 3.

1. Which of the curves in the figure above represents a modulation transfer function (MTF)?
   a. A
   b. B
   c. C
   d. D
   e. E

2. Which of the curves in the figure represents the digital image receptor radiation response?
   a. A
   b. B
   c. C
   d. D
   e. E

3. Which of the curves in the figure represents a line spread function?
   a. A
   b. B
   c. C
   d. D
   e. E

4. Spatial frequency consists of units of:
   a. Line length
   b. Line pair
   c. Line pair/millimeter
   d. Millimeter
   e. Millimeter/line pair

5. As an object gets smaller, which of the following gets bigger?
   a. ll
   b. lp
   c. lp/mm
   d. mm
   e. mm/lp

6. A breast microcalcification is spherical and 300 μm in diameter. What is the spatial frequency of this tissue object?
   a. 0.5 lp/mm
   b. 0.6 lp/mm
   c. 1.0 lp/mm
   d. 1.7 lp/mm
   e. 2.7 lp/mm

7. A calcified lung nodule measures 1 cm. What spatial frequency does this represent?
   a. 0.05 lp/mm
   b. 0.1 lp/mm
   c. 0.5 lp/mm
   d. 1.0 lp/mm
   e. 5.0 lp/mm

8. The best a multislice computed tomography imaging system can image is 1.5 lp/mm. This represents an object of what size?
   a. 125 µm
   b. 333 µm
   c. 400 µm
   d. 550 µm
   e. 675 µm

9. Modulation Transfer Function (MTF) for a digital imaging system has a cutoff spatial frequency of 5 lp/mm. What is the pixel size?
   a. 10 µm
   b. 25 µm
   c. 50 µm
   d. 100 µm
   e. 200 µm

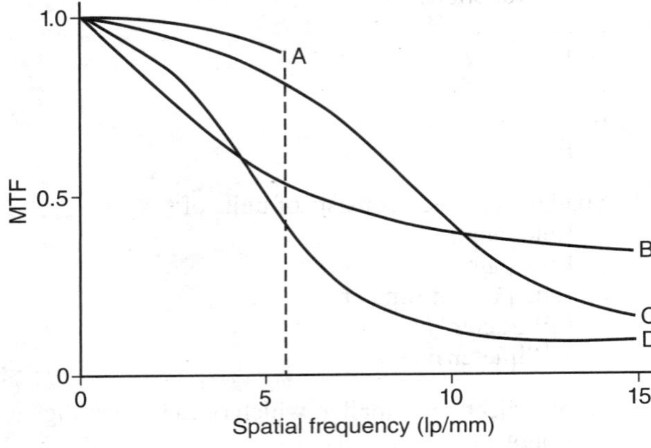

Use the figure above to answer Questions 10 and 11.

10. Which of the curves in the figure above represents the best spatial resolution?
    a. A
    b. B
    c. C
    d. D

11. Which of the curves in the figure represents digital radiography?
    a. A
    b. B
    c. C
    d. D

Worksheet 13-2 Contrast Resolution Contrast Detail

Digital radiography has poorer spatial resolution than previous imaging processes, such as screen-film imaging. However digital radiography has superior contrast resolution and is important for image quality and interpretation. Contrast resolution results in the ability to distinguish many shades of gray on an image.

The number of gray levels that an imaging system can produce is called **dynamic range**. The human visual system can see perhaps 30 shades of gray. Today's digital imaging systems are capable of rendering up to 65,536 shades of gray (16 bits), all visible with postprocessing of the image.

One method for evaluating the relative spatial and contrast resolutions of imaging systems is the contrast-detail curve. The use of such a curve shows that spatial resolution is determined by the MTF of the imaging system; contrast resolution is limited by the noise of the system.

EXERCISES

1. Which of the following reduces contrast resolution?
   a. Detective quantum efficiency (DQE)
   b. kVp
   c. mAs
   d. Modulation Transfer Function (MTF)
   e. Noise

2. If the dynamic range of a magnetic resonance imaging system is 12 bits, how many shades of gray are present?
   a. 1024
   b. 2048
   c. 4096
   d. 8192
   e. 16,384

3. Contrast resolution in computed tomography is superior compared to other x-ray systems because of:
   a. Collimation
   b. Detective Quantum Efficiency (DQE)
   c. The range of tissue values
   d. Modulation Transfer Function (MTF)
   e. Spiral motion

4. "Technique creep" is an attempt to reduce patient radiation dose by instituting:
   a. Increased DQE
   b. Increased kVp and reduced mAs
   c. Increased mAs and reduced kVp
   d. Increased mAs and reduced noise
   e. No repeats

5. The digital radiographic imaging repeat rate due to poor radiographic technique should not exceed:
   a. 0%
   b. 1%
   c. 5%
   d. 10%
   e. 25%

6. Detective quantum efficiency (DQE) is a measure of:
   a. Contrast resolution
   b. Digital data file size
   c. Image noise
   d. Spatial resolution
   e. X-ray absorption

7. The principal advantage of digital radiography:
   a. Contrast resolution
   b. Easier patient positioning
   c. Fewer repeats
   d. Less noise
   e. Reduced radiographic technique

8. The x-ray beam incident on the image receptor compared with the one incident on the patient:
   a. Has higher energy
   b. Has higher mAs
   c. Has the same energy
   d. Has lower energy
   e. Has poorer image receptor absorption

9. The dynamic range of a typical digital imaging system is:
   a. 4096
   b. 30
   c. 1000
   d. 3000
   e. 65,536

10. Why do digital imaging systems have a higher modulation transfer function (MTF) at low spatial frequencies?
    a. Better contrast resolution
    b. Fewer repeats
    c. Higher detective quantum efficiency (DQE)
    d. Less kVp dependence
    e. Lower patient dose

11. The postprocessing method used to allow us to see all shades of gray in an image is referred to as:
    a. Detective quantum efficiency (DQE)
    b. Window and level
    c. Spatial resolution
    d. Contrast detail
    e. Technique optimization

12. Spatial resolution in digital imaging systems is determined principally by:
    a. The type of image receptor
    b. Grid size
    c. Collimation
    d. Focal-spot size
    e. Pixel size

Worksheet 14-1 Exposure Time

$$\text{mAs} = \text{mA} \times \text{s}$$

$$\text{Therefore exposure time(s)} = \frac{\text{mAs}}{\text{mA}}$$

To get the greatest benefit from this worksheet, try to solve the problems mentally, without writing them down or using a calculator. If you need additional help with math techniques, turn to the Math Tutor section of this workbook.

EXERCISES

1. If the required technique is 2.5 mAs and the mA station selected is 100 mA, what is the required exposure time?
   a. 10 ms
   b. 15 ms
   c. 25 ms
   d. 75 ms
   e. 125 ms
2. If the required technique is 7.5 mAs and the mA station selected is 150 mA, what is the required exposure time?
   a. 10 ms
   b. 20 ms
   c. 30 ms
   d. 40 ms
   e. 50 ms
3. If the required technique is 20 mAs and the mA station selected is 300 mA, what is the required exposure time?
   a. 15 ms
   b. 67 ms
   c. 87 ms
   d. 133 ms
   e. 140 ms
4. If the required technique is 80 mAs and the mA station selected is 400 mA, what is the required exposure time?
   a. 15 ms
   b. 50 ms
   c. 150 ms
   d. 200 ms
   e. 350 ms
5. If the required technique is 33 mAs and the mA station selected is 100 mA, what is the required exposure time?
   a. 17 ms
   b. 33 ms
   c. 170 ms
   d. 330 ms
   e. 670 ms
6. If the required technique is 20 mAs and the mA station selected is 400 mA, what is the required exposure time?
   a. 5 ms
   b. 10 ms
   c. 20 ms
   d. 33 ms
   e. 50 ms
7. If the required technique is 25 mAs and the mA station selected is 200 mA, what is the required exposure time?
   a. 125 ms
   b. 150 ms
   c. 225 ms
   d. 275 ms
   e. 325 ms
8. If the required technique is 60 mAs and the mA station selected is 300 mA, what is the required exposure time?
   a. 100 ms
   b. 200 ms
   c. 300 ms
   d. 400 ms
   e. 600 ms
9. If the required technique is 240 mAs and the mA station selected is 400 mA, what is the required exposure time?
   a. 600 ms
   b. 900 ms
   c. 1200 ms
   d. 1500 ms
   e. 1800 ms

10. If the required technique is 5 mAs and the mA station selected is 100 mA, what is the required exposure time?
    a. 5 ms
    b. 15 ms
    c. 25 ms
    d. 50 ms
    e. 100 ms

11. If the required technique is 40 mAs and the mA station selected is 200 mA, what is the required exposure time?
    a. 25 ms
    b. 50 ms
    c. 100 ms
    d. 150 ms
    e. 200 ms

12. If the required technique is 5 mAs and the mA station selected is 300 mA, what is the required exposure time?
    a. 10 ms
    b. 17 ms
    c. 34 ms
    d. 50 ms
    e. 67 ms

13. If the required technique is 1.6 mAs and the mA station selected is 100 mA, what is the required exposure time?
    a. 16 ms
    b. 17 ms
    c. 34 ms
    d. 40 ms
    e. 50 ms

14. If the required technique is 1.25 mAs and the mA station selected is 50 mA, what is the required exposure time?
    a. 10 ms
    b. 25 ms
    c. 75 ms
    d. 125 ms
    e. 250 ms

15. If the required technique is 15 mAs and the mA station selected is 100 mA, what is the required exposure time?
    a. 15 ms
    b. 25 ms
    c. 50 ms
    d. 150 ms
    e. 250 ms

16. If the required technique is 120 mAs and the mA station selected is 300 mA, what is the required exposure time?
    a. 100 ms
    b. 200 ms
    c. 300 ms
    d. 400 ms
    e. 500 ms

17. If the required technique is 1.25 mAs and the mA station selected is 100 mA, what is the required exposure time?
    a. 1.25 ms
    b. 12.5 ms
    c. 25 ms
    d. 40 ms
    e. 50 ms

18. If the required technique is 4 mAs and the mA station selected is 200 mA, what is the required exposure time?
    a. 2 ms
    b. 4 ms
    c. 10 ms
    d. 20 ms
    e. 40 ms

19. If the required technique is 12.5 mAs and the mA station selected is 100 mA, what is the required exposure time?
    a. 1.25 ms
    b. 5 ms
    c. 12.5 ms
    d. 25 ms
    e. 125 ms

Worksheet 14-2
Adjusting for Change in Distance

Use the "square law" to find a new mAs that will compensate for a change in distance. While the **inverse square law** is used to predict radiation intensity, the square law is used to compensate radiographic technique so that radiation intensity is maintained constant when source-to-image receptor distance (SID) changes.

The square law:

$$\frac{mAs_2}{mAs_1} = \frac{(SID_2)^2}{(SID_1)^2}$$

where mAs_1 is the original mAs used at SID_1 (the original SID), and mAs_2 is the new mAs needed to maintain equal intensity if the SID is changed to SID_2.

EXERCISES

1. When radiographic technique is changed from 30 mAs, 100 cm SID, to 75 cm SID, what should be the new mAs?
   a. 17 mAs
   b. 20 mAs
   c. 24 mAs
   d. 30 mAs
   e. 32 mAs

2. When radiographic technique is changed from 12.5 mAs, 100 cm SID, to 150 cm SID, what should be the new mAs?
   a. 18 mAs
   b. 20 mAs
   c. 22 mAs
   d. 28 mAs
   e. 32 mAs

3. When radiographic technique is changed from 10 mAs, 100 cm SID, to 180 cm SID, what should be the new mAs?
   a. 20 mAs
   b. 26 mAs
   c. 30 mAs
   d. 32 mAs
   e. 36 mAs

4. When radiographic technique is changed from 5 mAs, 100 cm SID, to 240 cm SID, what should be the new mAs?
   a. 14 mAs
   b. 19 mAs
   c. 24 mAs
   d. 29 mAs
   e. 36 mAs

5. When radiographic technique is changed from 48 mAs, 80 cm SID, to 90 cm SID, what should be the new mAs?
   a. 51 mAs
   b. 55 mAs
   c. 59 mAs
   d. 61 mAs
   e. 71 mAs

6. When radiographic technique is changed from 22.5 mAs, 100 cm SID, to 200 cm SID, what should be the new mAs?
   a. 50 mAs
   b. 70 mAs
   c. 78 mAs
   d. 84 mAs
   e. 90 mAs

7. When radiographic technique is changed from 36 mAs, 150 cm SID, to 113 cm SID, what should be the new mAs?
   a. 20 mAs
   b. 26 mAs
   c. 30 mAs
   d. 38 mAs
   e. 48 mAs

8. When radiographic technique is changed from 10 mAs, 150 cm SID, to 225 cm SID, what should be the new mAs?
   a. 17 mAs
   b. 22.5 mAs
   c. 27.5 mAs
   d. 32.5 mAs
   e. 36 mAs

9. When radiographic technique is changed from 60 mAs, 70 kVp, 150 cm SID, to 113 cm SID, what should be the new mAs?
   a. 34 mAs
   b. 86 mAs
   c. 96 mAs
   d. 102 mAs
   e. 116 mAs

10. A posteroanterior chest examination done at 100 cm SID tabletop technique requires 1.5 mAs. What is the required mAs when testing is conducted with a dedicated chest imaging system with a fixed 180 cm SID?
   a. 1 mAs
   b. 2 mAs
   c. 3 mAs
   d. 5 mAs
   e. 10 mAs

11. If the dedicated chest room in Question 10 was designed for a fixed SID of 300 cm, what would be the required mAs?
   a. 1 mAs
   b. 3 mAs
   c. 5 mAs
   d. 13.5 mAs
   e. 20 mAs

12. A dedicated mammography imaging system has a fixed SID of 55 cm and normal technique calls for 200 mAs. If this system is replaced by a 75-cm mammography imaging system, what will be the approximate new mAs?
   a. 200 mAs
   b. 275 mAs
   c. 325 mAs
   d. 375 mAs
   e. 500 mAs

13. In magnification radiography, when the object is placed equidistant between the source and the image receptor, the size of the image will be:
   a. 1.33 times the object size
   b. 2.0 times object size
   c. 4 times the object size
   d. One-half the object size
   e. The same size as the object

14. A radiographic technique that would ensure visibility of detail for a cervical spine examination is:
   a. Increasing the OID
   b. Reducing the SID
   c. Reducing the SSD
   d. Selecting the large focal spot
   e. Using a beam-restricting device

15. The major disadvantage to magnification radiography is increased:
   a. Artifacts
   b. Blur
   c. Cost
   d. Noise
   e. Patient radiation dose

16. If SID is increased from 50 to 75 cm, what should happen to exposure time?
   a. Increase by $\frac{4}{9}$
   b. Increase by $\frac{2}{3}$
   c. No change
   d. Increase by $\frac{3}{2}$
   e. Increase by $\frac{9}{4}$

17. An x-ray field that is 25 × 30 cm at 100 cm SID is projected at 180 cm SID. The area of the projected field is:
   a. 750 cm^2
   b. 1350 cm^2
   c. 2430 cm^2
   d. 13,500 cm^2
   e. 22,600 cm^2

Worksheet 14-3
Characteristics of the Imaging System

Proper radiographic exposure must consider several variable characteristics of the x-ray imaging system. Perhaps the most important characteristic is the type of high-voltage generator incorporated into the imaging system. In general, compared with single-phase generators, full-wave rectified and more complex waveform generators require a lower kVp and lower mAs to produce acceptable radiographs. The radiologic technologist has no control over this characteristic.

Essentially all x-ray imaging systems now have selectable added filtration. The choices of added filtration available to the radiologic technologist usually range from 0 to 4 mm Al, resulting in total filtration of 1.5 to 5.5 mm Al.

EXERCISES

1. Which of the following is a popular focal-spot combination (small/large) for a dedicated mammography imaging system?
   a. 0.05 mm/0.2 mm
   b. 0.1 mm/0.3 mm
   c. 0.1 mm/3 mm
   d. 0.3 mm/1.0 mm
   e. 0.3 m/1.2 mm

2. The approximate filtration of the x-ray beam contributed by the light-localizing collimator is:
   a. 0.1 mm Al
   b. 0.5 mm Al
   c. 1.0 mm Al
   d. 2.0 mm Al
   e. 3.0 mm Al

3. The radiologic technologist cannot change the type of high-voltage generator used because:
   a. A change can be made only by the medical physicist.
   b. It is fixed at the time of purchase.
   c. Only the radiologic engineer can make that change.
   d. Only the radiologist can make that change.
   e. The service engineer determines this at installation.

4. Compared with half-wave rectification for a fixed exposure time:
   a. Full-wave rectification will have four times the number of pulses.
   b. High frequency will have six times the number of pulses.
   c. Three-phase will have at least six times the number of pulses.
   d. Three-phase will have at least 12 times the number of pulses.
   e. Three-phase will have four times the number of pulses.

5. The principal advantage of a large focal spot compared with a small focal spot is:
   a. Spatial resolution is enhanced.
   b. Contrast resolution is improved.
   c. Faster image receptors can be used.
   d. Voltage ripple is reduced.
   e. A greater number of x-rays can be produced.

6. An acceptable radiograph is made with a large focal spot. If the examination were repeated with the small focal spot using the same technique:
   a. Patient dose would be lower.
   b. The image would be darker.
   c. The image would be lighter.
   d. The image would be sharper.
   e. The image would have better contrast.

7. General purpose x-ray tubes usually have inherent filtration of:
   a. 0.1 mm Al
   b. 0.5 mm Al
   c. 1.0 mm Al
   d. 2.0 mm Al
   e. 3.0 mm Al

8. Which of the following has the least voltage ripple?
   a. High frequency
   b. Single-phase, full-wave
   c. Single-phase, half-wave
   d. Three-phase, six-pulse
   e. Three-phase, 12-pulse

9. Three-phase rectified power has which of the following?
   a. Three pulses per cycle
   b. Six pulses per cycle
   c. Nine pulses per cycle
   d. 15 pulses per cycle
   e. 18 pulses per cycle

10. An acceptable radiograph is made with a large focal spot. If the examination were repeated with the small focal spot:
    a. kVp should be reduced.
    b. mAs and kVp should be increased.
    c. mAs and kVp should be reduced.
    d. mAs should be reduced.
    e. No technique change is required.

11. The principal advantage of a small focal spot compared with a large focal spot is:
    a. Better detail
    b. Use of faster image receptors
    c. Higher heat capacity
    d. Reduced voltage ripple
    e. Production of a greater number of x-rays

12. An acceptable radiograph is made with 1.0 mm Al added filtration and a small focal spot. If the examination were repeated with 3.0 mm Al added filtration, what would be the most likely technique change?
    a. Increase kVp
    b. Increase kVp and mAs
    c. Decrease mAs
    d. Increase SID
    e. Use the larger focal-spot size

13. An acceptable radiograph is produced with a half-wave rectified x-ray imaging system. If the examination is repeated on a full-wave imaging system, what should be changed?
    a. Exposure time
    b. kVp
    c. mAs
    d. Object-to-image receptor distance
    e. SID

14. An acceptable radiograph is made with 1.0 mm Al added filtration. If the examination were repeated with 3.0 mm Al added filtration and appropriate technique changes made:
    a. Image blur would be reduced.
    b. Image contrast would improve.
    c. Patient dose would be reduced.
    d. Spatial resolution would improve.
    e. Such an exposure would not be possible.

15. An acceptable radiograph is made with a single-phase generator. If a repeat examination is performed with a three-phase generator, what technique change should be made?
    a. Increase kVp and mAs
    b. Increase mAs
    c. No change is required
    d. Reduce kVp
    e. Reduce kVp and mAs

16. What is the principal advantage of high-frequency generators?
    a. Better spatial resolution
    b. Enhanced radiation quality
    c. Increased radiation quantity and quality
    d. Reduced radiation quantity
    e. Reduced radiation quantity and quality

Worksheet 14-4
Magnification Radiography

In general radiography, overlying and underlying tissues are superimposed. In tomography, these tissues are blurred.

Magnification radiography requires an increase in object-to-image receptor distance (OID) to produce a magnified image. The degree of magnification is given by the magnification factor (MF).

$$MF = \frac{\text{Image size}}{\text{Object size}} = \frac{SID}{SOD}$$

Magnification radiography works best with a small x-ray tube focal spot. It usually can be performed without radiographic grids, yet it still results in a somewhat higher patient dose.

EXERCISES

1. Adequate magnification radiography requires that which of the following must have a large value?
   a. Focal spot
   b. OID
   c. SID
   d. SOD
   e. SSD

2. Magnification radiography normally is used to image what type of structure?
   a. High-contrast
   b. Large
   c. Low-contrast
   d. Moving
   e. Small

3. The MF is equal to which of the following?
   a. SID + OID
   b. SID ÷ SOD
   c. SOD + OID
   d. SOD ÷ SID
   e. SSD × SID

4. For magnification cerebral angiography, which of the following focal-spot sizes would be best?
   a. 0.3 mm
   b. 0.6 mm
   c. 1.0 mm
   d. 2.0 mm
   e. 10 mm

5. The major disadvantage of magnification radiography is increased:
   a. Artifacts
   b. Blur
   c. Cost
   d. Noise
   e. Patient dose

6. If the MF is 1.5 and the image size is 9 cm, what is the object size?
   a. 3 cm
   b. 6 cm
   c. 12 cm
   d. 13.5 cm
   e. 15 cm

Worksheet 15-1
Production of Scatter Radiation

Scatter radiation results from Compton interaction with patient tissue and reduces image contrast. Three principal factors influence the quantity of scatter radiation. Two of these can be manipulated by the radiologic technologist.

- **Kilovoltage (kVp):** Increasing kVp also increases the proportion of scatter radiation because the Compton effect predominates at higher energies.
- **Field size:** Scatter radiation increases with increasing field size because more tissue is exposed.
- **Patient thickness:** Scatter radiation increases as patient thickness increases. X-ray beam collimation and tissue compression reduce scatter radiation and therefore improve image contrast.

EXERCISES

1. Remnant x-rays are those that:
   a. Are absorbed within the patient
   b. Do not interact with the patient or the image receptor
   c. Exit the patient
   d. Interact with the patient and are scattered away
   e. Scatter back toward the source

2. Which of the following factors that affect scatter radiation can be controlled by the radiologic technologist?
   a. Added filtration
   b. Field size
   c. Inherent filtration
   d. mAs
   e. Patient thickness

3. As kVp increases, scatter radiation will:
   a. Decrease because of less Compton interaction
   b. Decrease because of less photoelectric interaction
   c. Increase because of more Compton interaction
   d. Increase because of more photoelectric interaction
   e. Remain unchanged

4. What is the approximate percentage of x-rays that are transmitted through a patient?
   a. 0.1%
   b. 1%
   c. 5%
   d. 10%
   e. 20%

5. At high kVp (e.g., 125 kVp), most x-rays are:
   a. Backscattered
   b. Not transmitted through the body
   c. Remnant x-rays
   d. Transmitted through the body with interaction
   e. Transmitted through the body without interaction

6. When kVp is increased with a compensating reduction in mAs, which of the following is reduced?
   a. Magnification
   b. Patient dose
   c. Remnant radiation
   d. Scatter proportion
   e. Spatial resolution

7. As field size is increased, scatter radiation:
   a. Increases
   b. Is reduced
   c. Is removed
   d. Is reversed
   e. Remains constant

8. Which of the following is not a device designed to reduce the level of scatter radiation that reaches the image receptor?
   a. A beam restrictor
   b. A collimator
   c. A compression device
   d. A diaphragm
   e. A test pattern

9. Scatter radiation reduces radiographic quality by changing:
   a. Blurring
   b. Contrast
   c. Distortion
   d. Mass density
   e. Beam intensity

10. X-rays that the technologist would like to have interact with the image receptor are those that are:
    a. Absorbed in the body
    b. Attenuated in the body
    c. High energy
    d. Scattered in the body
    e. Transmitted in the body

11. As kVp is increased from 70 to 80:
    a. Contrast resolution will improve.
    b. The mAs must be increased.
    c. The source-to-image receptor distance (SID) must be increased.
    d. There will be a higher proportion of scatter radiation.
    e. There will be a lower proportion of scatter radiation.

12. Image-forming x-rays consist of which type that emerge from the patient in the direction of the image receptor?
    a. Absorbed x-rays
    b. Backscattered x-rays
    c. Emitted x-rays
    d. Intercepted x-rays
    e. Transmitted x-rays

13. As kVp increases from 70 to 90, if all other factors remain constant:
    a. Contrast resolution will improve.
    b. The number of absorbed x-rays will decrease.
    c. The number of transmitted x-rays will decrease.
    d. The ratio of absorbed to transmitted x-rays will increase.
    e. The ratio of scattered to transmitted x-rays will increase.

14. What increases as the field size of the x-ray beam increases?
    a. Heel effect
    b. kVp
    c. mAs
    d. Scatter radiation
    e. Total filtration

15. In general, as the thickness of the anatomy for which radiographs are made increases:
    a. Contrast resolution improves.
    b. kVp is increased.
    c. mAs is increased.
    d. Patient exposure is unaffected.
    e. Total filtration is increased.

16. Which of the following processes is most responsible for the production of scatter radiation?
    a. Bremsstrahlung interaction
    b. Characteristic interaction
    c. Compton effect
    d. Photoelectric effect
    e. Transmission

Worksheet 15-2
Control of Scatter Radiation

Beam-restricting devices are used in radiology to limit the volume of tissue irradiated to reduce patient dose and scatter radiation. Three types of beam-restricting devices exist:

- **Aperture diaphragm:** A fixed-aperture device that consists of a lead or lead-lined metal diaphragm attached to the head of the x-ray tube.
- **Cones and cylinders:** Fixed-aperture devices that consist of an extended metal structure attached to the x-ray tube head.
- **Variable-aperture collimator:** A device that consists of two or more pairs of lead shutters that are independently adjustable. Square or rectangular fields are possible, and the x-ray field can be illuminated by a coincidence light field.
- **Positive beam–limiting (PBL)** devices automatically collimate to the image receptor size.

EXERCISES

1. Which of the following is not a beam-restricting device?
   a. A cone
   b. A PBL device
   c. A variable-aperture collimator
   d. Added filtration

2. An aperture diaphragm should allow x-rays to expose an area:
   a. Equal to the image receptor
   b. Just larger than the image receptor
   c. Just smaller than the image receptor
   d. That varies according to patient size
   e. That varies according to technique

3. When an aperture diaphragm is used:
   a. A PBL device is required.
   b. Added filtration should be increased.
   c. Grid cutoff can occur if the diaphragm is not properly positioned.
   d. Technique should be enhanced.
   e. X-ray field cutoff can occur if the diaphragm is not properly positioned.

4. In a light-localizing, variable-aperture collimator:
   a. Added filtration is required.
   b. Equipped with a PBL device, light field illumination is unnecessary.
   c. If the lightbulb burns out, the graduated scale on the adjusting mechanism can be used.
   d. It is not necessary that the crosshairs in the light beam be centered.
   e. Periodic checks of x-ray beam and light field coincidence are necessary.

5. Which of the following is the simplest of all beam-restricting devices?
   a. A fluoroscopic collimator
   b. A radiographic cone
   c. An aluminum filter
   d. An aperture diaphragm
   e. PBL

6. Which of the following devices is normally designed to limit off-focus radiation?
   a. Added filtration
   b. First-stage shutters of a variable-aperture collimator
   c. Fixed-aperture circular diaphragms
   d. Fixed-aperture rectangular diaphragms
   e. Second-stage shutters of a variable-aperture collimator

7. Off-focus radiation:
   a. Consists of scattered electrons
   b. Consists of scattered electrons and x-rays
   c. Improves image quality
   d. Increases patient dose
   e. Results when projectile electrons do not strike the focal spot

8. Which of the following is a beam-restricting device?
   a. 2.5 mm Al added filtration
   b. A cone without an integral diaphragm
   c. A rectangular film mask on a viewbox
   d. A fluoroscopic spot-film device
   e. PBL

9. Cone cutting:
   a. Is useful in high-kVp examinations
   b. Is useful in low-kVp examinations
   c. Occurs when the axis of the cone, tube, and image receptor are not aligned
   d. Occurs when the edge of the cone intercepts the scattered x-ray beam
   e. Occurs when the tip of the cone is too close to the patient

10. If a fixed-aperture, rectangular, beam-restricting device is used:
   a. Added filtration is unnecessary.
   b. An unexposed border should be visible on all four sides of the radiograph.
   c. An unexposed border should be visible on at least two sides of the radiograph.
   d. PBL must be used.
   e. The central axis of the aperture diaphragm must be centered somewhere on the image receptor.

11. A properly designed, light-localizing, variable-aperture collimator:
   a. Concentrates off-focus radiation onto the image receptor
   b. Is designed to enhance off-focus radiation
   c. Needs no added filtration
   d. Requires light field/x-ray beam coincidence
   e. Will have field-defining shutters of aluminum

12. Radiographic cones and cylinders are used principally to reduce which of the following?
   a. Beam quality
   b. Off-focus radiation
   c. Scatter radiation
   d. The need for added filtration
   e. The required radiographic technique

13. Which of the following are the two general types of devices designed to control scatter radiation?
   a. Filtration and beam restrictors
   b. Filtration and image masks
   c. Grids and beam restrictors
   d. Grids and filtration
   e. Image masks and beam restrictors

14. When a diaphragm is used:
   a. A 1-cm unexposed border should be visible on all sides.
   b. A 1-cm unexposed border should be visible on two sides.
   c. A 3-cm unexposed border should be visible on at least three sides.
   d. Added filtration must be increased.
   e. An unexposed border is not necessary.

15. PBL stands for which of the following?
   a. Photon beam level
   b. Photon beam limitation
   c. Photon border level
   d. Positive beam level
   e. Positive beam limitation

16. A diaphragm is machined to just match the image receptor size. If an unexposed border is required on the radiograph, the diaphragm opening will:
   a. Have to be enlarged.
   b. Have to be reduced.
   c. More information is required before a change can be determined.
   d. Remain the same.
   e. Require additional filtration.

17. An aperture diaphragm is designed for a 25-cm × 30-cm image. If the SID is 100 cm and the source-to-diaphragm distance is 10 cm, what size should the opening of the diaphragm be?
   a. 2.0 cm × 2.5 cm
   b. 2.0 cm × 3.0 cm
   c. 2.5 cm × 3.0 cm
   d. 2.5 cm × 3.5 cm
   e. 3.0 cm × 3.5 cm

Worksheet 15-3 Radiographic Grids

X-rays that leave a patient and are incident on the image receptor are called image-forming radiation. There are two basic components of image-forming radiation: (1) those x-rays that have passed directly through the patient without interaction and (2) those x-rays that have been scattered within the patient. Only the x-rays that are not significantly scattered carry useful diagnostic information to the image receptor.

Scattered x-rays are the result of Compton interaction. Because the image receptor is not capable of distinguishing primary x-rays from scattered x-rays, it will image a scattered x-ray as having come directly from the x-ray source when, in fact, its direction was from the tissue from which it was scattered. This scattered radiation reduces image contrast.

The main device used to intercept scattered radiation is the grid. There are two principal characteristics of grid construction: (1) grid ratio is the thickness of the grid (the height of the grid strip) divided by the width of the interspace material and (2) grid frequency is the number of grid strips per inch or per centimeter.

EXERCISES

1. The principal reason for using a grid is to:
   a. Enhance differential absorption
   b. Improve image contrast
   c. Improve spatial resolution
   d. Reduce patient dose
   e. Remove remnant radiation

2. Which of the following materials would be most radiolucent?
   a. Aluminum
   b. Carbon fiber
   c. Copper
   d. Iodine
   e. Lead

3. Which of the following is the most important grid characteristic?
   a. Grid frequency
   b. Grid height
   c. Grid mass
   d. Grid ratio
   e. Grid weight

4. In a grid that has lead strips 0.5 mm apart and 4 mm high, the grid ratio is:
   a. 4:1
   b. 6:1
   c. 8:1
   d. 12:1
   e. 16:1

5. A grid has the following characteristics: grid ratio = 10:1; grid height = 4.5 mm; grid strip width = 40 μm; and interspace width = 450 μm. What is the grid frequency?
   a. 20 lines/cm
   b. 22 lines/cm
   c. 40 lines/cm
   d. 45 lines/cm
   e. 60 lines/cm

6. If only scatter radiation reached the image receptor:
   a. Image contrast would be very high.
   b. Image contrast would be very low.
   c. Image receptor speed would be very high.
   d. Image receptor speed would be very low.
   e. Spatial resolution would be improved.

7. In the design of a radiographic grid, which of the following must be true?
   a. The added filtration must be aluminum.
   b. The grid strips are radiolucent.
   c. The grid strips are radiotransparent.
   d. The interspace material is radiolucent.
   e. The interspace material is radiopaque.

8. Grids are principally effective in attenuating which of the following?
   a. All remnant radiation
   b. Photoelectrons
   c. Transmitted x-rays
   d. X-rays after Compton interaction
   e. X-rays after photoelectric interaction

9. If the interspace dimension is constant, increasing the grid ratio will:
   a. Make the grid lighter
   b. Make the grid thicker
   c. Reduce grid mass
   d. Require less grid strip material
   e. Require less interspace material

10. As grid frequency increases:
   a. Grid mass is usually decreased.
   b. The grid ratio is reduced if the thickness of the grid remains constant.
   c. The interspace width becomes thinner if the width of the grid strip remains constant.
   d. The number of grid strips per centimeter decreases.
   e. The patient dose is reduced.

11. Which of the following would be the most acceptable grid strip material from the standpoint of x-ray attenuation?
   a. Barium
   b. Copper
   c. Iodine
   d. Tungsten
   e. Uranium

12. Which of the following will not improve image contrast?
   a. A decrease in kVp
   b. Collimating the x-ray beam
   c. The use of a grid
   d. The use of added filtration
   e. The use of positive-beam limitation (PBL)

13. Grids with a high ratio are:
   a. Easier to manufacture than those with a low ratio
   b. More effective than those with a low ratio
   c. Most effective at low kVp
   d. Produced by increasing grid strip width
   e. Produced by increasing interspace width

14. The efficiency of a grid for reducing scatter radiation is related principally to which of the following?
   a. Grid frequency
   b. Grid interspace
   c. Grid mass
   d. Grid radius
   e. Grid ratio

15. Radiographic grids:
   a. Can be placed anywhere between the source and the image receptor
   b. Can be placed between the patient and the image receptor
   c. Can be placed between the source and the patient
   d. Must be placed between the patient and the image receptor
   e. Must be placed between the source and the patient

16. The construct of a radiographic grid:
   a. Has an aluminum cover for filtration
   b. Has an aluminum cover to reduce scatter radiation
   c. Incorporates aluminum or copper as the grid strip material
   d. Incorporates high-Z interspace material
   e. Is easier to achieve with an aluminum interspace than with plastic fiber

17. Use of which of the following will reduce radiographic contrast?
   a. Collimators
   b. Filtration
   c. Grids
   d. Aperture diaphragm
   e. PBL

Worksheet 15-4 Measuring Grid Performance

The principal function of a radiographic grid is to absorb scattered radiation from the image-forming x-ray beam before it reaches the image receptor. If scattered radiation does reach the image receptor, the image contrast is reduced. The function of radiographic grids is to increase image contrast.

The higher the grid ratio and the higher the grid frequency, the greater the image contrast. The principal measure of grid performance is the contrast improvement factor, K:

$$K = \frac{\text{Radiographic contrast with a grid}}{\text{Radiographic contrast without a grid}}$$

Another measure of grid performance is selectivity:

$$\text{Selectivity} = \frac{\text{Transmitted primary x-rays}}{\text{Transmitted scattered x-rays}}$$

Both the contrast improvement factor and selectivity depend on the characteristics of the x-ray beam and the characteristics of the grid. However, the contrast improvement factor depends more on the characteristics of the x-ray beam, whereas selectivity depends more on the construction of the grid.

EXERCISES

1. Which of the following is the least important indicator of grid performance?
   a. Contrast improvement factor
   b. Grid frequency
   c. Grid mass
   d. Grid strip height
   e. Grid ratio

2. As the grid ratio increases, there is also an increase in which of the following?
   a. Spatial frequency
   b. Grid mass
   c. Spatial resolution
   d. Grid radius
   e. Width of interspace material

3. In general, the selectivity of a grid depends principally on which of the following?
   a. Contrast improvement factor
   b. Focal length
   c. Grid frequency
   d. Grid mass
   e. Grid radius

4. Radiographic grids with high contrast improvement usually:
   a. Are low-ratio grids
   b. Improve contrast resolution
   c. Improve spatial resolution
   d. Reduce patient dose
   e. Transmit more scatter radiation

5. A radiograph is made at 76 kVp and 25 mAs without a grid. If an 8:1 ratio grid is added, the mAs required then would be approximately:
   a. 25 mAs
   b. 50 mAs
   c. 100 mAs
   d. 150 mAs
   e. 300 mAs

6. Which of the following is the simplest type of grid?
   a. Crossed grid
   b. Focused grid
   c. High-ratio grid
   d. Linear grid
   e. Zero frequency grid

7. The undesirable absorption of image-forming x-rays by a grid is called:
   a. Anode heel effect
   b. Grid cutoff
   c. Malpositioned grid
   d. Primary beam scatter
   e. Upside-down grid

8. Which of the following would be included in the three major classifications of moving grids?
   a. Crossed grid
   b. Focused grid
   c. Linear grid
   d. Reciprocating grid
   e. Zero frequency grid

9. If one had two grids whose characteristics were unknown, but grid B weighed twice as much as grid A, one might conclude that grid B would have:
   a. A higher contrast improvement factor
   b. A greater mass effect
   c. A lower grid frequency
   d. A lower grid ratio
   e. A lower selectivity

10. Focused grids:
    a. Cut off the four edges of an image if placed too close to the source
    b. Cut off two edges of an image if placed too far from the tube
    c. Do not move
    d. Reduce the amount of scatter radiation that reaches the image receptor
    e. Reduce the radiation exposure to the patient compared with no grid

11. One factor that does not affect the percentage of scatter radiation that reaches the image receptor is:
    a. Grid mass
    b. Grid ratio
    c. kVp
    d. mAs
    e. Patient thickness

12. The Bucky factor increases with which of the following?
    a. Decreasing contrast improvement factor
    b. Decreasing grid ratio
    c. Increasing interspace width
    d. Increasing x-ray quality
    e. Increasing x-ray quantity

13. Which of the following would principally reduce the production of scatter radiation?
    a. A decrease in field size
    b. A decrease in SID
    c. An increase in SSD
    d. Use of a filter
    e. Use of a grid

14. Radiographic grids:
    a. Have reduced selectivity as the mass is increased
    b. May have aluminum step wedges incorporated into them
    c. Must include a filter
    d. Usually have contrast improvement factors from 0 to 1.0
    e. Usually have grid ratios between 5:1 and 16:1

15. A crossed radiographic grid:
    a. Allows considerable positioning latitude compared with linear grids
    b. Has a contrast improvement factor equal to a linear grid of equal ratio
    c. It is said to have a grid ratio of 10:1; therefore it consists of two 5:1 linear grids
    d. Must be used for tomography
    e. Reduces scatter radiation along two axes

16. Which of the following is a disadvantage of moving grids?
    a. They may produce motion blur.
    b. They may result in decreased magnification.
    c. They require higher grid frequency.
    d. They require a higher grid ratio.
    e. They require thinner strips.

Worksheet 15-5
Types of Grids
Use of Grids
Grid Selection

If the construction and performance characteristics of a grid are known and understood, grid selection and use will be more accurate. Selection of a grid usually requires that one specify the type of grid (parallel, crossed, focused, or moving), the ratio of the grid, and the grid frequency.

Such selection is made on the basis of the types of radiographic examination to be performed. If grid lines are objectionable, moving grids should be used.

Cerebral angiography often requires crossed grids so that contrast is maximized for imaging small-vessel details. Low-kVp techniques usually demand low-ratio grids, and high-kVp techniques usually require high-ratio grids. For general purpose radiographic rooms, focused grids with ratios of approximately 8:1 to 12:1 usually are used.

Focused grids are normally preferred to parallel grids because with parallel grids, grid cutoff can occur.

$$\text{Distance to grid cutoff} = \frac{\text{Source-to-image receptor distance}}{\text{Grid ratio}}$$

EXERCISES

1. Which of the following is not a grid positioning error?
   a. Air-gap grid
   b. Lateral decentering
   c. Off-center grid
   d. Off-focus grid
   e. Off-level grid

2. In the design of radiographic techniques, the most common practice is to use which of the following?
   a. A crossed grid
   b. A focused moving grid
   c. A focused stationary grid
   d. A parallel moving grid
   e. A parallel stationary grid

3. Grids generally:
   a. Must be cleaned annually
   b. Require faster image receptors
   c. Require lower mAs
   d. Require periodic replacement because of radiation fatigue
   e. Result in increased patient dose

4. When comparable radiographs are produced, which of the following combinations will result in the lowest patient dose?
   a. High kVp and high-ratio grids
   b. High kVp and low-ratio grids
   c. High kVp and no grid
   d. Low kVp and high-ratio grids
   e. Low kVp and low-ratio grids

5. Grid cutoff:
   a. Is measured by the Bucky factor
   b. Is more pronounced with high-ratio grids
   c. Is more pronounced with low-ratio grids
   d. Never occurs with focused grids
   e. Occurs only with focused grids

6. Air-gap technique:
   a. Increases the Bucky factor
   b. Reduces contrast by absorption of scattered radiation in the air
   c. Requires that the grid and the film must be separated by at least 30 cm
   d. Results in approximately the same patient dose as nongrid techniques
   e. Results in image magnification

7. If radiographic grids are used and the technique is compensated, patient exposure:
   a. Increases with increasing grid ratio
   b. Increases with increasing kVp
   c. Is independent of grid frequency
   d. Is independent of grid mass
   e. Remains unchanged from that with nongrid techniques

8. Bedside examinations require a wide range of SIDs. Which of the following parallel grids would be most likely to produce grid cutoff?
   a. 5:1
   b. 6:1
   c. 8:1
   d. 12:1
   e. 16:1
9. In general, which of the following has the greatest contrast improvement factor?
   a. Crossed grids
   b. Focused grids
   c. Moving grids
   d. Parallel grids
   e. Zero grids
10. Which of the following is an undesirable characteristic of linear grids compared with focused grids?
    a. Higher Bucky factor
    b. Increased patient dose
    c. Lower grid frequencies
    d. Lower grid ratios
    e. More grid cutoff
11. What is the result of replacing an 8:1 grid with a 12:1 grid?
    a. Greater positioning latitude
    b. Higher patient dose
    c. Less contrast
    d. Less spatial resolution
    e. Lower patient dose
12. When air-gap radiography is performed:
    a. A high-ratio grid must be used.
    b. A low-ratio grid must be used.
    c. Contrast resolution is improved.
    d. Patient dose is increased.
    e. The heel effect is accentuated.
13. As grid frequency increases:
    a. Grid mass is usually reduced.
    b. The grid ratio will be reduced if the thickness of the grid remains constant.
    c. The interspace width becomes thinner if the width of the grid strip remains constant.
    d. The number of grid strips per centimeter increases.
    e. The patient dose is reduced.
14. Radiographic grids:
    a. Have reduced selectivity as the mass is increased.
    b. May have aluminum step wedges incorporated into them.
    c. Must also include a filter.
    d. Usually have contrast improvement factors from 0 to 1.0.
    e. Usually have grid ratios between 5:1 and 16:1.
15. Bedside examinations require a wide range of SIDs. Which of the following linear grids would be most likely to produce grid cutoff?
    a. 5:1
    b. 6:1
    c. 8:1
    d. 12:1
    e. 16:1

Worksheet 16-1 Image Descriptors

Image quality has many descriptive terms to express the exactness of representation of the patient's anatomy on a medical image. High-quality images are required so that radiologists can make accurate interpretations and diagnoses. To produce high-quality images, radiographers apply knowledge of the interrelated categories of image quality: spatial resolution, contrast resolution, geometric factors, and subject factors. Each of these descriptors influences the quality of a medical image, and each is under the control of the radiologic technologists.

EXERCISES

1. What two factors affect image magnification?
   a. Spatial resolution and contrast resolution
   b. Preprocessing and postprocessing
   c. Source-to-image receptor distance (SID) and lateral distance
   d. SID and object-to-image receptor distance (OID)
   e. Source-to-skin distance (SSD) and OID

2. What is the magnification factor (MF)?
   a. OID/SID
   b. SID/OID
   c. SID/SOD
   d. SOD/OID
   e. SOD/SID

3. When assessing image quality, which of the following would be considered a *subject factor?*
   a. Atomic number
   b. Distortion
   c. Dynamic range
   d. Pixel size
   e. Postprocessing

4. Which of the following is most difficult to image because of low object contrast?
   a. Breast microcalcifications
   b. Liver-spleen
   c. Lung nodules
   d. Meniscal tear
   e. Ventricles

5. Regarding image perception and interpretation, what is the most important image descriptor?
   a. Artifacts
   b. Contrast resolution
   c. Noise
   d. Pixel size
   e. Spatial resolution

6. When describing image quality, all of the following apply except:
   a. Contrast resolution
   b. Digital device display (DDD)
   c. Geometric factors
   d. Spatial resolution
   e. Subject factors

7. A microcalcification measures 400 μm on a full field mammogram obtained at an SID of 70 cm. With compression the OID is estimated to be 2 cm. What is the true size of the microcalcification?
   a. 402 μm
   b. 407 μm
   c. 412 μm
   d. 417 μm
   e. 422 μm

8. When the source-to-object distance (SOD) cannot be estimated, the object size can use which expression?
   a. Object size = Image size (OID/SID)
   b. Object size = Image size (OID/SOD)
   c. Object size = Image size (SID/SOD)
   d. Object size = Image size (SOD/SID)
   e. Object size = (SOD/SID)/(OID/SOD)

9. The term *image sharpness* is most closely related to the physics term
   a. Contrast resolution
   b. Dynamic range
   c. Postprocessing
   d. Preprocessing
   e. Spatial resolution

10. What is the largest source of radiographic noise?
    a. Artifacts
    b. Compton scatter radiation
    c. Focal spot size
    d. Motion
    e. Object size

11. Considering all of the medical imaging modalities, which has the best contrast resolution?
    a. Computed tomography (CT)
    b. Diagnostic ultrasound
    c. Digital breast tomosynthesis
    d. Magnetic resonance imaging (MRI)
    e. Positron emission tomography (PET)

12. Which of the following medical imaging modalities is most frequently clinically employed?
    a. CT
    b. Diagnostic ultrasound
    c. Digital radiography
    d. MRI
    e. PET

13. What is the anatomic mass size when the image size is 8.5 cm and is made at 100 cm SID? The OID is estimated to be 20 cm.
    a. 8.5 cm
    b. 8.6 cm
    c. 6.8 cm
    d. 9.1 cm
    e. 9.3 cm

14. What is the MF?
    a. Anterior-posterior (AP) size/lateral size
    b. Image size/object size
    c. Large focal spot size/small focal spot size
    d. Lateral size/AP size
    e. Object size/image size

15. When assessing image quality, which of the following would be considered a geometric factor?
    a. Dynamic range
    b. Image blur
    c. Mass density
    d. Patient motion
    e. Pixel size

16. Use of which of the following is a good way to reduce quantum noise?
    a. DDD
    b. Low mAs, low kVp
    c. High mAs, low kVp
    d. High ratio grid
    e. Low mAs, high kVp

17. Which of the following is particularly important when considering contrast resolution?
    a. Contrast scale
    b. Image size matters
    c. Noise scale
    d. Object size matters
    e. Single-photon emission computed tomography versus PET

18. What principal characteristic of medical imaging determines spatial resolution?
    a. Focal spot size
    b. Image noise
    c. Pixel size
    d. Spatial contrast
    e. Spatial frequency

19. We associate a high-contrast image with which of the following?
    a. High spatial resolution
    b. Large focal spot size
    c. Large object size
    d. High kVp
    e. Low kVp

20. When assessing image quality, which of the following would be considered an image receptor factor?
    a. Atomic number
    b. Image blur
    c. Object contrast
    d. Patient motion
    e. Pixel size

Worksheet 16-2
Image Quality Tools

Radiologic technologists normally have the tools available to produce high-quality radiographic images. Proper patient preparation, the selection of proper image receptors, and proper radiographic technique are complex, related concepts.

For any given radiographic examination, each of these factors must be properly interpreted and applied. A small change in one may require a compensating change in another. Patient positioning, image receptors, and the selection of technique factors are critical parts of image quality.

EXERCISES

1. Which of the following examinations can be performed without consideration of the heel effect?
   a. Abdomen
   b. Anterior-posterior (AP) thoracic spine
   c. Femur
   d. Lateral skull
   e. Posterior-anterior (PA) chest

2. What is the principal advantage of using an image receptor having a large matrix size?
   a. Reduced blur
   b. Reduced patient motion
   c. Improved spatial resolution
   d. Reduced postprocessing
   e. Reduced preprocessing

3. What characteristic of radiographic quality is improved by using reduced x-ray exposure time?
   a. Anatomic shape
   b. Higher effective atomic number
   c. Increased mass density
   d. Increased tissue thickness
   e. Motion blur

4. Radiographic contrast is related to the product of what image characteristics?
   a. Attenuation and absorption
   b. Contrast resolution and spatial resolution
   c. Image preprocessing and image postprocessing
   d. Scatter radiation and attenuation
   e. Subject contrast and image receptor contrast

5. A 0.3 mm effective focal spot is used to image a 400 μm breast microcalcification. The SID is 70 cm, and the microcalcification is 1 cm from the image receptor. What will be the focal spot blur?
   a. 4.8 μm
   b. 5.3 μm
   c. 5.8 μm
   d. 6.3 μm
   e. 6.8 μm

6. Which of the following imaging modalities comes closest to providing a three-dimensional image?
   a. Computed tomography
   b. Digital radiographic tomosynthesis
   c. Doppler ultrasound
   d. Functional magnetic resonance imaging
   e. PET

7. What is the result on the image when an anatomic structure is not equally magnified?
   a. Blur
   b. Distortion
   c. Excess magnification
   d. Excess minification
   e. Minification

8. The radiologic technologist can minimize bothersome magnification by using a larger:
   a. OID
   b. Object-to-skin distance
   c. SID
   d. SOD
   e. SSD

9. What is the principal advantage of digital radiographic image receptors with small pixel size?
   a. Better contrast resolution
   b. Better spatial resolution
   c. Easier preprocessing
   d. Fewer digital artifacts
   e. Less image noise

10. Which of the following radiographic techniques should be engaged for a PA chest examination?
    a. Cathode to abdomen side
    b. Extensive postprocessing
    c. High kVp
    d. Low mAs
    e. Neglect preprocessing

11. Which of the following principally influences contrast resolution?
    a. Exposure time
    b. Motion blur
    c. Patient motion
    d. Postprocessing
    e. Preprocessing

12. Subject contrast affects image contrast through each of the following **except**:
    a. Atomic number (Z)
    b. Patient motion
    c. Postprocessing
    d. Tissue mass density
    e. Tissue thickness

13. What is the approximate pixel size in digital radiography?
    a. 50 μm
    b. 100 μm
    c. 175 μm
    d. 200 μm
    e. 300 μm

14. How can we best describe the effect of focal spot blur on an image?
    a. Relatively unimportant
    b. Results in elongation
    c. Results in foreshortening
    d. Results in larger pixel size
    e. Results in superposition

15. Image distortion depends on all of the following **except**:
    a. Focal spot size
    b. Object shape
    c. Object thickness
    d. OID
    e. SSD

16. Which of the following will **not** help to reduce motion blur?
    a. Increase dynamic range
    b. Increase SID
    c. Reduce OID
    d. Use a patient immobilization device
    e. Use short x-ray exposure time

17. What is the main advantage of increased kVp/reduced mAs when performing digital radiography?
    a. Reduced blur
    b. Reduced patient motion
    c. Reduced patient radiation dose
    d. Reduced postprocessing
    e. Reduced preprocessing

18. What is one of the consequences of the anode heel effect?
    a. Reduced focal spot blur on the anode side of the image
    b. Reduced focal spot blur on the cathode side of the image
    c. Reduced kVp on the cathode side of the image
    d. Reduced mAs on the cathode side of the image
    e. Reduced x-ray intensity on the cathode side of the image

19. Focal spot blur is equal to the product of effective focal spot size and
    a. OID/SOD
    b. SOD/OID
    c. SSD/OID
    d. SSD/SOD
    e. SSD + SOD

20. Image distortion occurs when:
    a. Proper postprocessing is not applied.
    b. Superposition is applied.
    c. The image plane and object plane are not parallel.
    d. The image plane and object plane are too far apart.
    e. The large focal spot is used.

Worksheet 17-1
Digital Radiographic Artifacts

An artifact is any feature on an image that does not truly represent tissue. Artifacts can interfere with diagnosis and obscure lesions or normal anatomy.

Digital imaging artifacts can be classified into three categories: image receptor artifacts, object artifacts, and processing artifacts. The radiologic technologist must be able to identify the source of an artifact.

Artifacts associated with pixel failure are easily identified but may be difficult to correct. Environmental radiation or previous exposure to computed radiography image receptors can produce ghost images. These are easily corrected. Preprocessing and postprocessing artifacts also are easily corrected, and the correction is automatic.

EXERCISES

1. Which of the following is ***not*** a digital imaging artifact?
   a. Alignment
   b. Collimation
   c. Density difference
   d. Image compression
   e. Partition

2. When does the radiologic technologist have to be concerned with processing artifacts?
   a. When compression is employed
   b. When image histograms are used
   c. When images are printed
   d. When partition is involved
   e. When software is corrupted

3. Ghost images can appear when:
   a. Radiation fatigue is present.
   b. Dust remains on the image receptor.
   c. A computed radiography (CR) image receptor has not been erased in 24 hours.
   d. A digital radiography (DR) image receptor is not completely read out.
   e. A proper quality control (QC) program is not instituted.

4. Which of the following should be presented to the radiologist for interpretation?
   a. For-compression image
   b. For-extrapolation image
   c. For-interpolation image
   d. For-presentation image
   e. For-processing image

5. Flat fielding is a preprocessing feature used to apply:
   a. Contrast resolution correction
   b. Geometric distortion correction
   c. An equalized response program
   d. Noise reduction algorithms
   e. Spatial resolution enhancement

6. What level of image compression is considered acceptable?
   a. 3:1
   b. 5:1
   c. 8:1
   d. 10:1
   e. 20:1

7. What does this artifact represent?

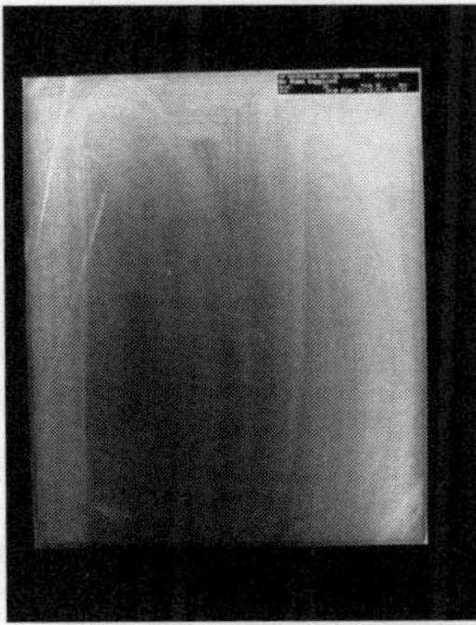

   a. Damaged imaging plate
   b. Debris on the imaging plate
   c. Inadequate erasure
   d. Postprocessing artifact
   e. Preprocessing artifact

8. What does this artifact represent?

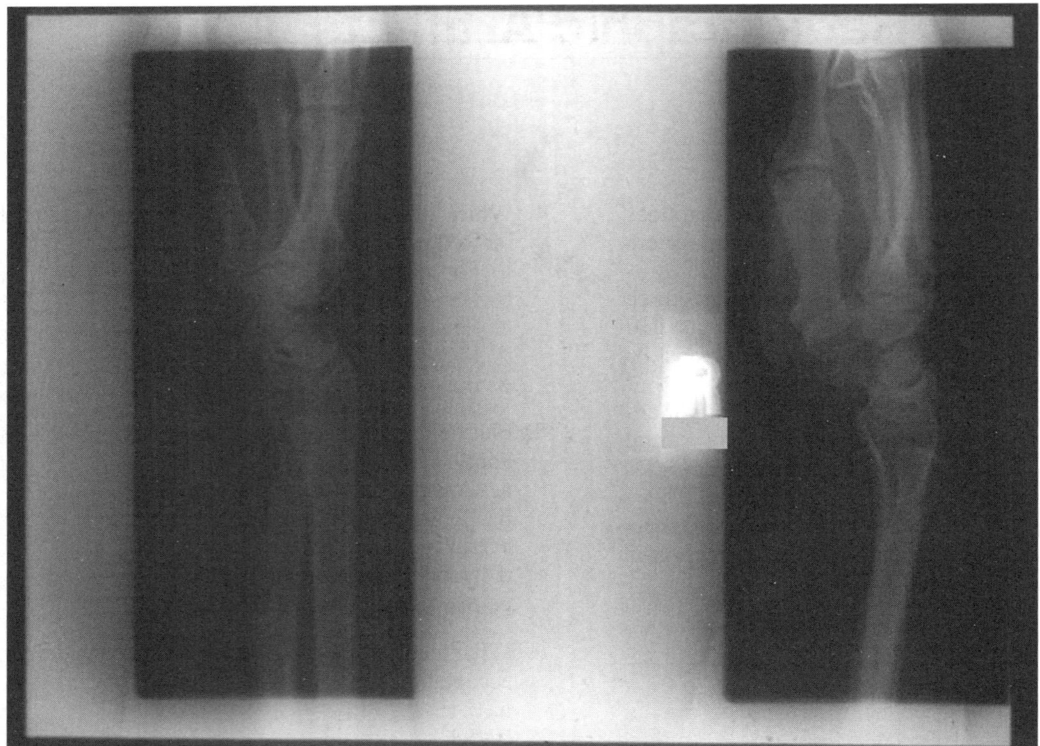

a. Inadequate erasure
b. Inappropriate reconstruction algorithm
c. Improper alignment
d. Improper collimation
e. Improper partition

9. What does this artifact represent?

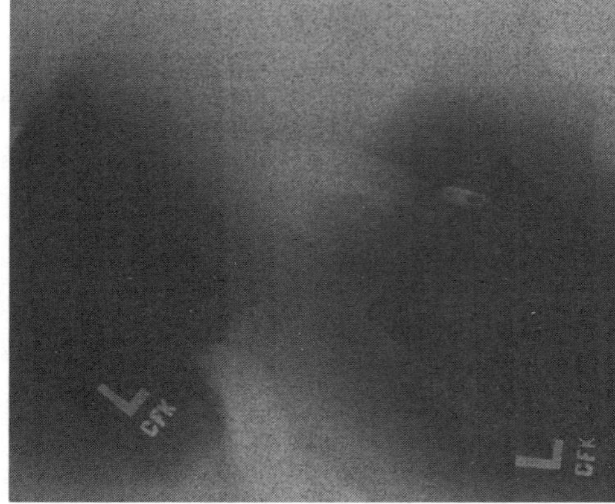

a. Ghost image
b. Improper collimation
c. Improper partition
d. Inadequate erasure
e. Preprocessing artifact

Worksheet 18-1 Mammography

Mammography is an examination of the breast with the use of low-energy x-rays. General-purpose x-ray imaging systems cannot be used successfully for mammography; a dedicated mammography x-ray imaging system is required.

Breast compression reduces motion blur, absorption blur, and patient dose, and improves spatial and contrast resolution.

The mammographic imaging system must be able to accurately produce x-rays in the range of 23 to 30 kVp. The system should have a molybdenum/rhodium-targeted x-ray tube. Such a tube emits radiation with K-characteristic x-rays at 19 and 23 keV, respectively. Because of the low filtration of mammography, the radiation exposure of the patient can be considerably higher than in general radiography.

EXERCISES

1. Low kVp is required for mammography because of which of the following?
   a. High mAs
   b. Patient positioning and compression
   c. Composition of breast tissue
   d. Type of image receptor used
   e. Varying thickness of breast tissue

2. When molybdenum is used for the x-ray tube target:
   a. kVp can be higher.
   b. mAs can be lower.
   c. No added filtration is required.
   d. No bremsstrahlung x-rays are produced.
   e. Useful characteristic x-rays are used.

3. If the cathode of the x-ray tube is positioned toward the chest wall during a cranial-caudal view:
   a. Absorption blur will be reduced.
   b. Exposure time will be reduced.
   c. Geometric blur will be greater toward the chest wall.
   d. The central ray will miss the breast.
   e. The image will display the entire breast.

4. In mammography, low kVp is selected to do which of the following?
   a. Improve spatial resolution
   b. Increase Compton absorption
   c. Increase photoelectric absorption
   d. Reduce patient dose
   e. Reduce skin reaction

5. When a mammogram taken at 23 kVp is compared with one taken at 28 kVp:
   a. For the same exit dose, the 28 kVp examination will require a higher entrance dose.
   b. If the mAs is constant, the exposure time will be less at 23 kVp.
   c. If the mAs is constant, the number of x-rays reaching the image receptor will be the same.
   d. Radiographic contrast will be enhanced at 28 kVp.
   e. The ratio of entrance dose to exit dose will be higher at 23 kVp.

6. The principal reason why molybdenum-targeted x-ray tubes are used in mammography is that molybdenum produces which of the following?
   a. A high atomic number
   b. A high melting point
   c. A higher heat capacity
   d. Useful bremsstrahlung x-rays
   e. Useful characteristic x-rays

7. Successful mammography cannot be done at 90 kVp because:
   a. Compton interactions are too few.
   b. Differential absorption is too low.
   c. Exposure time is too long.
   d. Patient dose is too high.
   e. X-ray tube heat is too great.

8. During mammography:
   a. More filtration is required.
   b. Radiographic contrast is low.
   c. The half-value layer is relatively low.
   d. Radiation quality is relatively high.
   e. X-ray transmission predominates.

9. Regarding the incidence of breast cancer in women, which of the following is *true?*
   a. Each year, about 10,000 new cases appear in the United States.
   b. It is on the decline.
   c. More than 80% of breast cancer results in death.
   d. The most critical decade is that of 30 to 40 years.
   e. The odds of developing breast cancer are 1 in 8.

10. In mammography, which of the following is *most* often responsible for image contrast?
    a. mAs
    b. kVp
    c. Tissue atomic number
    d. Tissue mass
    e. Tissue mass number

11. X-ray tube potential below 20 kVp is ***not*** used because:
    a. Characteristic x-rays are not produced.
    b. Compton interaction predominates.
    c. Generators are not available for such low voltage.
    d. There are no x-rays below 20 keV.
    e. X-ray penetration is not sufficient.

12. Why is SID reduced in mammography compared with conventional radiography?
    a. To decrease exposure time
    b. To decrease geometric unsharpness
    c. To improve differential absorption
    d. To improve spatial resolution
    e. To reduce patient dose

13. If an x-ray tube is positioned so that the anode is toward the chest wall during a cranial-caudad view:
    a. Image-forming x-rays will have more uniform intensity at the image receptor.
    b. Patient dose will be lower.
    c. Spatial resolution will be higher toward the nipple.
    d. Exposure time will be about one-half.
    e. Radiation exposure will be greater at the nipple than at the chest wall.

14. The principal reason why mammography is widely used is that:
    a. It is easy.
    b. It is inexpensive.
    c. t is reimbursable.
    d. The incidence of breast cancer is high.
    e. The radiation dose is low.

15. Which of the following target/filter combinations is *most* appropriate for screening mammography?
    a. Mo/Al
    b. Mo/Mo
    c. Rh/Mo
    d. W/Al
    e. W/Mo

16. Compression during mammography is necessary to do which of the following?
    a. Comfort the patient
    b. Increase OID
    c. Increase SID
    d. Reduce geometric blur
    e. Use the small focal spot

17. Mammography grids are designed to do which of the following?
    a. Decrease contrast
    b. Improve contrast
    c. Improve spatial resolution
    d. Reduce geometric blur
    e. Reduce patient dose

Worksheet 18-2
Quality Control Team
Quality Control Program

The purposes of a mammography quality control (QC) program are to produce the best possible diagnostic images through good equipment performance and to ensure that the patient receives the best available care with the least radiation exposure. QC falls under the larger umbrella of quality assurance (QA), which is an administrative program that ensures that all tasks of the QC team are carried out at the highest level. Continuous quality improvement is an extension of any QC/QA program and includes administrative protocols for the continuous improvement of mammographic quality.

The mammography QC team includes a radiologist, a medical physicist, and a mammographer. Radiologists oversee the QA program and track diagnostic results. Medical physicists examine and monitor the performance of imaging equipment, and they chart and record data to ensure compliance with the latest recommendations and standards. Mammographers perform many tests and evaluations that involve equipment, processing, and mammographic images.

EXERCISES

1. Which of the following describes the difference between Quality Control (QC) and Quality Assurance (QA)?
   a. QC deals with the performance of imaging apparatuses.
   b. QC defines the quality of the QA team.
   c. QC is focused on patient scheduling, examination, and reporting.
   d. QA is concerned principally with image processing.
   e. QA is the responsibility of the mammographer.

2. Who is principally responsible for the QC/QA program?
   a. Administrator
   b. Mammographer
   c. Medical physicist
   d. QC technologist
   e. Radiologist

3. CQI stands for which of the following?
   a. Cautious quality improvement
   b. Competent quality imaging
   c. Continuous quality improvement
   d. Controlled quality insistence
   e. None of the above

4. The assessment of glandular dose in mammography is principally the responsibility of which of the following staff members?
   a. Administrator
   b. Mammographer
   c. Medical physicist
   d. QC technologist
   e. Radiologist

5. The responsibilities of the medical physicist must be carried out at *least:*
   a. Daily
   b. Weekly
   c. Monthly
   d. Quarterly
   e. Annually

6. Which member of the mammography QC/QA team is principally responsible for daily QC/QA?
   a. Administrator
   b. Mammographer
   c. Medical physicist
   d. Patient
   e. Radiologist

7. The duties of the QC mammographer include the tasks that should be performed:
   a. Daily
   b. Daily and weekly
   c. Daily, weekly, and quarterly
   d. Daily, weekly, quarterly, and annually
   e. Daily, quarterly, and annually

Worksheet 19-1 Image Intensification

The image-intensifier tube was introduced to radiology in the 1950s for the principal purpose of reducing patient dose. The image-intensifier tube improves image quality and diagnostic accuracy.

The dose reduction produced by the image intensifier, called **brightness gain**, is the product of the geometric gain, or **minification**, and the **flux gain**.

Direct digital and solid-state flat-panel image receptors are beginning to completely replace the image-intensifier tube.

EXERCISES

1. Photoelectric emission:
   a. Is the emission of electrons from a heated wire
   b. Is the emission of electrons from an illuminated surface
   c. Is the emission of photons
   d. Occurs at the input phosphor of an image-intensifier tube
   e. Occurs at the output phosphor of an image-intensifier tube

2. At what stage of image-intensified fluoroscopy is the number of image-forming photons lowest?
   a. Entering the input phosphor
   b. Entering the photocathode
   c. Leaving the input phosphor
   d. Leaving the output phosphor
   e. Leaving the photocathode

3. Image-intensifier brightness gain increases with increasing:
   a. Flux gain
   b. kVp
   c. mA
   d. Output phosphor size
   e. Radiation exposure

4. When an image intensifier receives x-rays at the input phosphor, what is emitted at the output phosphor?
   a. Electrons
   b. Infrared light
   c. Ultraviolet light
   d. Visible light
   e. X-rays

5. Which of the following is the input phosphor of image intensifiers?
   a. Cadmium tungstate
   b. Calcium tungstate
   c. Cesium iodide
   d. Sodium iodide
   e. Zinc cadmium sulfide

6. Which of the following is the output phosphor of image intensifiers?
   a. Cadmium tungstate
   b. Calcium tungstate
   c. Cesium iodide
   d. Sodium iodide
   e. Zinc cadmium sulfide

7. The photocathode converts:
   a. Electrons into visible light
   b. Visible light into electrons
   c. Visible light into x-rays
   d. X-rays into electrons
   e. X-rays into visible light

8. Which of the following is the component of the image intensifier responsible for focusing the electron beam?
   a. Electrostatic lens
   b. Glass envelope
   c. Input phosphor
   d. Output phosphor
   e. Photocathode

9. The ability of an image intensifier to enhance image illumination is called:
   a. Automatic brightness
   b. Brightness gain
   c. Flux gain
   d. Illumination gain
   e. Minification gain

10. The minification gain of an image intensifier increases with increasing:
    a. Input phosphor size
    b. kVp
    c. mA
    d. Output phosphor size
    e. Tube voltage

11. Which of the following is a representative brightness gain for an image intensifier?
    a. 200
    b. 2000
    c. 20,000
    d. 200,000
    e. 2 million

12. If an image intensifier is described as a $^{25}/_{12}$ tube, $^{25}/_{12}$ refers to which of the following?
    a. Area of the input phosphor in square inches
    b. Diameter of the input phosphor in centimeters
    c. Diameter of the output phosphor in centimeters
    d. Radius of the input phosphor in inches
    e. Radius of the output phosphor in centimeters

13. When a multifocus image intensifier is operated in the magnification mode:
    a. A larger area of input phosphor is used.
    b. Contrast resolution is reduced.
    c. Patient dose is lower.
    d. Spatial resolution is reduced.
    e. The electron focal point is closer to the input phosphor.

14. An image that displays vignetting:
    a. Is dim around the periphery
    b. Is dim in the center
    c. Has higher contrast resolution
    d. Has higher spatial resolution
    e. Shows the barrel stays artifact

15. With a multifocus image intensifier in the magnification mode:
    a. Contrast resolution is reduced.
    b. Noise is increased.
    c. Patient dose is reduced.
    d. Spatial resolution is improved.
    e. Field of view is increased.

16. In a 10/7/5 image intensifier:
    a. Contrast resolution is best in the 10 mode.
    b. Spatial resolution is best in the 10 mode.
    c. The field of view is largest in the 10 mode.
    d. There are three different input phosphors.
    e. There are three different output phosphors.

17. An image intensifier has a 5-cm output phosphor and a 45-cm input phosphor. The brightness gain is 10,000. The flux gain is approximately:
    a. 10
    b. 80
    c. 120
    d. 1000
    e. 5000

18. Place the following in the proper sequence for image-intensified fluoroscopy:
    1. Electric signal to light
    2. Electrons to light
    3. Light to electric signal
    4. Light to electrons
    5. X-ray to light
    a. 1, 2, 3, 4, 5
    b. 2, 3, 4, 5, 1
    c. 3, 5, 2, 1, 4
    d. 5, 3, 1, 4, 2
    e. 5, 4, 2, 3, 1

19. Which of the following applies to the output phosphor?
    a. Electrons emitted
    b. Light absorbed
    c. Light emitted
    d. X-rays absorbed
    e. X-rays emitted

Worksheet 19-2
Image Monitoring

The fluoroscopic image produced at the output phosphor of an image-intensifier tube is the size of a postage stamp and cannot be viewed directly. This image is manipulated for viewing, or **monitoring**, with a closed-circuit television system. The output image of the image-intensifying tube is detected by a television camera tube, usually a **vidicon** or a charge-coupled device, and then is displayed on a television or a flat-panel monitor.

Such images can be monitored with an optically coupled cine camera that is usually restricted to use during specialized examinations, such as cardiac catheterization, but has mainly been replaced by digital imaging. If static images are required during the examination, they are made with an optically coupled spot-film camera.

EXERCISES

1. Vertical television resolution is limited principally by which of the following?
   a. Bandpass
   b. Field rate
   c. Frame rate
   d. Lines per frame
   e. Modulation

2. The electron beam in a television camera tube is produced by which of the following means?
   a. Electroemission
   b. Photoconduction
   c. Photoemission
   d. Thermionic emission
   e. Thermoluminescence

3. What is the camera tube most used in television fluoroscopy?
   a. Cesium iodide
   b. Electrons from light
   c. Minification
   d. Synchronized
   e. Vidicon

4. What is the photoemissive component of image-intensified fluoroscopy?
   a. Cesium iodide
   b. Electrons from light
   c. Minification
   d. Synchronized
   e. Vidicon

5. Which of the following is photoconductive?
   a. Electron gun
   b. Electrostatic grid
   c. Signal plate
   d. Target
   e. Window

6. What is the principal disadvantage of coupling the television camera to the image intensifier with the use of fiber optics?
   a. Cassette-loaded spot film cannot be used.
   b. Fragility is increased.
   c. Image noise is increased.
   d. Photospot camera cannot be used.
   e. Spatial resolution is reduced.

7. Which of the following refers to the image-intensifier input phosphor?
   a. Cesium iodide
   b. Electrons from light
   c. Minification
   d. Synchronized
   e. Vidicon

8. Which is a critical component in optically coupling an image intensifier with a photospot camera?
   a. Electrostatic lens
   b. Face plate
   c. Objective lens
   d. Signal plate
   e. Subjective lens

9. What is the *most* important component of a television monitor?
   a. Cathode ray tube
   b. Charge-coupled device
   c. Coupling device
   d. Electromagnetic coils
   e. Television camera tube

10. In an optical coupling arrangement, which is nearest the television camera?
    a. Beam splitter
    b. Camera lens
    c. Deflection coil
    d. Mirror
    e. Objective lens

11. What is the component of the television monitor in which the video signal is transformed into an image?
    a. Electron beam
    b. Electron gun
    c. Electrostatic grid
    d. Phosphor plate
    e. Target assembly

12. What is the electron beam of the television camera tube?
    a. A fan beam
    b. An area beam
    c. Blanked
    d. Collimated
    e. Modulated

13. One television frame is equivalent to which of the following?
    a. 17 ms
    b. 262½ lines
    c. 1024 lines
    d. One television field
    e. Two television fields

14. Fluoroscopic television operates at a frame rate of:
    a. 30 frames per second
    b. 60 frames per second
    c. 262½ frames per second
    d. 525 frames per second
    e. 1024 frames per second

15. Horizontal television resolution is limited principally by which of the following?
    a. Bandpass
    b. Field rate
    c. Frame rate
    d. Lines per frame
    e. Modulation

16. What is normally the weakest imaging link in television fluoroscopy?
    a. Image-intensifier tube
    b. Optical coupling device
    c. Spot-film device
    d. Television camera
    e. Television monitor

17. Common frame rates during cinefluorography are 15, 30, and 60 f/s because:
    a. Flicker is not observed at these rates.
    b. It is linked to patient dose.
    c. Of the frame rate requirement of the television camera tube.
    d. Of the frequency of the power supply.
    e. The film format requires it.

18. When the electron beam of the cathode ray tube (CRT) is blanked, it is:
    a. Demodulated
    b. In a vertical retrace
    c. In an active trace
    d. Modulated
    e. Turned on

19. What is the television camera tube component of image-intensified fluoroscopy?
    a. Cesium iodide
    b. Electrons from light
    c. Minification
    d. Synchronized
    e. Vidicon

Worksheet 19-3 Digital Fluoroscopy

Digital fluoroscopy has been developed as a replacement for some earlier angiographic procedures such as subtraction angiography. With digital fluoroscopy, such subtraction images are relatively easily and quickly produced, and postprocessing and manipulation of the image are possible.

In digital fluoroscopy, a high signal-to-noise ratio (SNR), high-resolution video system is coupled with a computer. The video signal is digitized, manipulated in the computer by one of several techniques, and finally displayed on the video monitor. Alternatively, solid-state flat-panel image receptors produce direct digital images.

EXERCISES

1. The principal reason for image integration is to:
   a. Improve contrast resolution
   b. Improve spatial resolution
   c. Reduce examination time
   d. Reduce image noise
   e. Reduce patient dose

2. The maximum frame acquisition rate in digital fluoroscopy is about:
   a. 1 frame per second
   b. 4 frames per second
   c. 10 frames per second
   d. 30 frames per second
   e. 60 frames per second

3. The SNR of a conventional TV camera tube is about:
   a. 100:1
   b. 200:1
   c. 1000:1
   d. 2000:1
   e. 5000:1

4. Compared with conventional fluoroscopy, digital fluoroscopy is conducted:
   a. At much higher x-ray tube current
   b. At much lower x-ray tube current
   c. With a different type of image intensifier
   d. With a different type of video monitor
   e. With higher-capacity x-ray tubes

5. Digital imaging systems can display images on a 1024 × 1024 matrix. How many pixels are present in such a matrix?
   a. 1000
   b. 1024
   c. 2048
   d. 1,048,576
   e. It depends on the grayscale.

6. A conventional radiograph is which of the following?
   a. A digital image
   b. A geometric image
   c. A linear image
   d. An analog image
   e. An exponential image

7. Which of the following components found in digital fluoroscopy is ***not*** found in conventional fluoroscopy?
   a. A video monitor
   b. An automatic brightness stabilizer
   c. An analog-to-digital converter (ADC)
   d. An image intensifier
   e. A source-to-image receptor distance indicator

8. During digital fluoroscopy, the image receptor is which of the following?
   a. Thin Film Transistor (TFT)
   b. Imaging plate
   c. The image-intensifier tube
   d. TV camera tube
   e. Video monitor

9. A principal advantage of digital fluoroscopy over conventional fluoroscopy for subtraction studies is:
   a. Contrast enhancement
   b. Examination speed
   c. Less contrast material
   d. Low patient dose
   e. Noise enhancement

10. The approximate pixel size for a 12-in. image-intensifier tube and a 256 reconstruction matrix is:
    a. 0.4 mm
    b. 0.8 mm
    c. 1.0 mm
    d. 2.5 mm
    e. 4 mm

11. During digital fluoroscopy:
    a. Both cine and spot film modes can be used.
    b. Neither cine nor spot film modes can be used.
    c. The x-ray beam is continuous and at high mA.
    d. The x-ray beam is continuous and at low mA.
    e. The x-ray beam is pulsed.

12. Digital fluoroscopy is conducted:
    a. At relatively low mA
    b. In the progressive TV mode
    c. With a large field of view
    d. With low patient dose
    e. With low signal-to-noise ratio (SNR)

13. How many video monitors are required for digital fluoroscopy?
    a. None
    b. 1
    c. 2
    d. 3
    e. 4

14. The time-interval difference mode is best used for which of the following?
    a. Dynamic studies
    b. Extremities
    c. High-dose examinations
    d. Large fields
    e. Long exposure times

15. Reregistration of an image is used to do which of the following?
    a. Correct any error in patient identification
    b. Correct for motion
    c. Increase edge enhancement
    d. Reduce noise
    e. Reduce patient dose

16. The combination of temporal subtraction and energy subtraction techniques is called:
    a. Enhanced subtraction
    b. Hybrid subtraction
    c. No subtraction
    d. Radiographic subtraction
    e. Resonance subtraction

17. The minimum acceptable TV signal to noise ratio (SNR) for digital fluoroscopy is:
    a. 100:1
    b. 200:1
    c. 1000:1
    d. 2000:1
    e. 5000:1

18. Interrogation time:
    a. Is the time spent questioning the patient
    b. Is the time needed to switch off the x-ray tube
    c. Is the time needed to switch on the x-ray tube
    d. Is the total exposure time
    e. Refers to the total examination time

19. A digital imaging system with a dynamic range of 2^{10} will be able to reproduce how many shades of gray?
    a. 32
    b. 256
    c. 512
    d. 1024
    e. 4096

20. An advantage of temporal subtraction over energy subtraction angiography is:
    a. Motion artifacts
    b. Higher patient dose
    c. Increased spatial resolution
    d. Higher contrast at lower dose
    e. More types of subtraction are possible.

21. An advantage of digital imaging over conventional imaging is which of the following?
    a. Increased latitude
    b. Increased resolution
    c. Postprocessing
    d. Reduced noise
    e. Limited resolution

22. A pixel is a:
    a. Matrix of numbers
    b. Range of numbers
    c. Three-dimensional digital image cell
    d. Two-dimensional digital image cell
    e. Unit of fluoroscopy dose

23. Between the TV camera and the computer of a digital fluoroscopic system is a/an:
    a. Analog-to-digital converter (ADC)
    b. Digital-to-analog converter
    c. Image-intensifier tube
    d. Image storage device
    e. Second video monitor

24. The mask image is usually the:
    a. First image
    b. Image at the peak of contrast
    c. Image just preceding contrast
    d. Last contrast image
    e. Last image

25. As one integrates video frames in digital fluoroscopy:
    a. Image noise is lower.
    b. Patient dose increases.
    c. Spatial resolution is improved.
    d. The signal-to-noise ratio (SNR) increases.
    e. Video noise is louder.

26. Which of the following components is uniquely essential to digital fluoroscopy?
    a. Analog-to-digital converter (ADC)
    b. Cathode Ray Tube (CRT)
    c. High-frequency generator
    d. TV camera pickup tube
    e. TV monitor

27. A misregistration artifact:
    a. Cannot be corrected or compensated
    b. Is not really an artifact
    c. Occurs when a patient moves
    d. Requires more hardware than is usually available
    e. Usually follows a change in kVp

28. Remasking:
    a. Can correct for patient motion
    b. Reduces spatial resolution
    c. Requires a change in kVp
    d. Requires a repeat examination
    e. Will increase patient dose

29. A matrix of what size can be held by 10 bytes of memory?
    a. 256 × 256
    b. 512 × 512
    c. 1024 × 1024
    d. 2084 × 2084
    e. 4096 × 4096

30. A 7-bit pixel can display how many shades of gray?
    a. 7
    b. 49
    c. 64
    d. 128
    e. 256

31. The idea behind digital subtraction angiography is:
    a. To decrease patient dose
    b. To see bone better
    c. To image vessels
    d. To increase signal-to-noise ratio (SNR)
    e. To decrease noise

32. How many numbers can be stored in 7 bits?
    a. 64
    b. 128
    c. 256
    d. 512
    e. 1024

33. How many bits are required to display 512 shades of gray?
    a. 5
    b. 6
    c. 7
    d. 8
    e. 9

34. How many shades of gray are possible in a pixel of size 2^{10}?
    a. 64
    b. 128
    c. 256
    d. 512
    e. 1024

35. The standard contrast material used in digital subtraction angiography is:
    a. Cesium
    b. Barium
    c. Gadolinium
    d. Sodium
    e. Iodine

36. If the same amount of imaging time occurs, compared to the dose in conventional fluoroscopy, the dose in digital fluoroscopy is:
    a. Higher
    b. Lower
    c. About the same
    d. It depends.
    e. None of the above

37. Which of the following is ***not*** an advantage of charge-coupled devices (CCDs) with regard to medical imaging?
    a. High signal-to-noise ratio (SNR)
    b. Low patient dose
    c. High spatial resolution
    d. Low cost
    e. Linear response

38. Reregistration of the mask involves:
    a. Acquiring more images
    b. Increasing patient dose
    c. Shifting image pixels
    d. Injecting more contrast
    e. Significant computation time

39. The k-edge for iodine is what energy?
    a. 16 keV
    b. 74 kVp
    c. 53 keV
    d. 33 keV
    e. 90 keV

40. During 5 minutes of digital fluoroscopy, a typical dose is:
    a. 200 mGy
    b. 5 mGy
    c. 200 mSv
    d. 500 mGy
    e. 500 mSv

41. Which of the following is *not* an advantage of flat-panel image receptors over charge-coupled devices (CCDs) coupled to image intensifiers in digital fluoroscopy?
    a. Distortion-free images
    b. Higher spatial resolution
    c. Constant image quality
    d. Improved contrast resolution
    e. High detective quantum efficiency (DQE)

Worksheet 20-1
Types of Procedures
Basic Principles
IR Suite

IR stands for *interventional radiography*. Radiographers who have passed the American Registry of Radiologic Technologists examination for cardiovascular and interventional radiography have the letters (CV) in their credentials.

Angiography refers to methods of imaging contrast-filled vessels. Vascular imaging and therapeutic intervention through vessels require a special suite equipped with advanced radiographic and fluoroscopic imaging systems. Special guidewires and catheters are used in interventional radiology to access the vascular network without surgery. Different catheter tips are designed to access specific arteries.

Charge-coupled devices (CCDs) are rapidly replacing the television camera tube as the image recorder. CCDs are photosensitive silicon chips that can be used anywhere that light will be converted to a digital video image. The advantages of CCDs for IR are many and include high spatial resolution, lack of spatial distortion, a linear response, lower patient dose, and the lack of warm-up and maintenance requirements.

EXERCISES

1. The term *angiography* refers to which of the following?
   a. Contrast examinations of arteries
   b. Contrast examinations of veins
   c. Contrast examinations of vessels
   d. Examination of brain vessels
   e. Examination of leg vessels

2. Transbrachial select coronary angiography refers to the examination of which of the following?
   a. Angiointerventional radiography
   b. Angioplasty
   c. Coronary arteries through an artery in the arm
   d. Coronary arteries through an artery in the leg
   e. The brachial artery

3. What is the principal reason to use guidewires in cardiovascular angiography and interventional radiology?
   a. Better visualization under fluoroscopy
   b. Ease of entry at the puncture site
   c. Safe introduction of the catheter into the vessel
   d. Visualization of arteries
   e. Visualization of veins

4. What is the approximate length of a conventional guidewire?
   a. 50 cm
   b. 100 cm
   c. 145 cm
   d. 200 cm
   e. 300 cm

5. To prevent clotting of blood within the catheter, what is the normal procedure?
   a. Saline flush
   b. Water flush
   c. Aspirin administration
   d. Heparinized saline flush
   e. Catheter occlusion

6. For vascular studies, the most often used radiopaque contrast medium is based on which of the following?
   a. Air
   b. Barium
   c. Calcium
   d. Iodine
   e. Gadolinium

7. After angiography:
   a. A physical examination is necessary to assess the patient's medical history for allergies and other conditions.
   b. Manual compression on the femoral site is not necessary once the catheter is removed.
   c. The patient usually can be released immediately.
   d. The patient is instructed to remain immobile for several hours.
   e. The patient is visited by the radiologist to establish rapport.

8. What does *osmolality* refer to when applied to contrast media?
   a. Atomic number of the media
   b. Concentration of ions in the media
   c. Mass density of the media
   d. Risk of the media
   e. Viscosity of the media

9. What is the principal complication of transfemoral angiography?
   a. Blood loss
   b. Hemorrhage of the puncture site
   c. Oxygen deprivation
   d. Patient anxiety
   e. Vessel collapse

10. Which of the following is an interventional procedure that would be conducted in an IR suite?
    a. Arteriography
    b. Arthrography
    c. Cardiac catheterization
    d. Myelography
    e. Stent placement

11. In an IR suite, a door between the operating console and the examination room:
    a. Is a protective barrier
    b. Is not required
    c. Must be double-hinged
    d. Must be double-wide
    e. Should accommodate a stretcher

12. Which of the following is a minimum requirement for an IR x-ray tube?
    a. 0.3-mm small focal spot
    b. 5-cm diameter anode
    c. 80-kW power rating
    d. 300,000-kHU anode heat capacity
    e. Molybdenum-targeted anode

13. For the spatial resolution requirements of the magnification of small vessels, the focal spot must be:
    a. No smaller than 0.3 mm
    b. No larger than 0.3 mm
    c. No smaller than 0.5 mm
    d. No larger than 0.5 mm
    e. None of the above

14. What is a characteristic of an IR x-ray tube?
    a. Large target angle
    b. Small-diameter anode disc
    c. Small target angle
    d. 50-kW power rating
    e. 300,000-kHU anode heat capacity

15. If an aortogram is performed with a 0.3-mm focal spot and source-to-image receptor distance (SID) of 100 cm, and the artery is 15 cm from the image receptor, what is the magnification factor?
    a. 0.85
    b. 1.08
    c. 1.10
    d. 1.18
    e. 1.25

Worksheet 21-1 Principles of Operation of CT

Computed tomography (CT) represents one of the most important developments in medical imaging of the 20th century. The development of slip-ring technology and high-frequency generators promoted the introduction of helical CT. This was followed by multi-slice CT for faster imaging of a larger tissue volume.

The CT imaging system has three principal sections: the gantry, the operating console, and the computer. The gantry assembly includes a high-voltage generator, an x-ray tube, a detector array, and the patient couch.

EXERCISES

1. A CT imaging system produces which type of image?
   a. Axial
   b. Biaxial
   c. Fulcrum plane
   d. Longitudinal
   e. Transverse

2. In its simplest configuration, the CT imaging system consists of an x-ray source and which of the following?
   a. A detector
   b. A selenium plate
   c. A video display terminal
   d. An image intensifier
   e. An x-ray beam collimator

3. Which of the following is characteristic of first-generation CT imaging systems?
   a. A pencil x-ray beam
   b. A selenium or film image receptor
   c. Multiple sources and multiple detectors
   d. Rotate-only geometry
   e. Slip rings

4. CT imaging systems incorporate:
   a. Charged electrostatic plates
   b. High-frequency radiographic grids
   c. Light-localizing, variable-aperture collimators
   d. Automatic brightness control
   e. A gantry

5. Sensitivity profile in CT is determined principally by the:
   a. Bow-tie filter
   b. Pre-detector collimator
   c. Pre-patient collimator
   d. Reconstruction algorithm
   e. Ramp function

6. Spatial resolution for CT imaging systems is approximately:
   a. 1 cm
   b. 10 cm
   c. 100 mm
   d. 1 mm
   e. 10 mm

7. Second-generation CT imaging systems:
   a. Have a multiple detector array
   b. Have rotate-rotate geometry
   c. Require imaging speeds from 1 to 5 minutes
   d. Require special patient preparation
   e. Use increments of 1 degree per view

8. Third-generation CT imaging systems have which of the following?
   a. Multiple-detector, area-beam geometry
   b. Rotate-rotate geometry
   c. Rotate-translate geometry
   d. Single-detector, fan-beam geometry
   e. Translate-translate geometry

9. Fourth-generation CT imaging systems:
   a. Are faster than third-generation CT imaging systems
   b. Have rotate-rotate geometry
   c. Incorporate area-beam geometry
   d. May use selenium as the image receptor
   e. Require pre-patient collimation

10. Which of the following subsystems would normally be associated with the gantry assembly?
   a. Image postprocessing
   b. The algorithms
   c. The detector array
   d. The physician's viewing console
   e. The software

11. Which of the following has been used as a detector in a CT imaging system?
   a. Bismuth germanate
   b. $CaWO_4$
   c. High-pressure air
   d. Selenium
   e. Silver halide

12. A comparison of scintillation and gas-filled detectors shows that:
    a. Both have approximately the same total detection efficiency.
    b. Both rely heavily on Compton interaction.
    c. Only scintillation detectors require pre-patient collimation.
    d. The gas-filled detectors have higher intrinsic efficiency.
    e. The scintillation detectors have higher detection efficiency.

13. In a CT imaging system, pre-patient collimation:
    a. Controls pixel size
    b. Controls scatter radiation that reaches the detector
    c. Determines image noise
    d. Determines image contrast
    e. Determines slice thickness

14. The translate-rotate mode:
    a. Collects data only during the rotate portion
    b. Describes both first- and second-generation CT imaging systems
    c. Requires higher heat capacity x-ray tubes
    d. Requires only solid-state detectors
    e. Results in imaging times as short as 1 s

15. Each translation of a source detector assembly produces which of the following?
    a. A matrix
    b. A pixel
    c. A projection
    d. A voxel
    e. An image

16. Slice thickness can also be expressed as which of the following?
    a. Dose profile
    b. Low-contrast profile
    c. Resolution profile
    d. Sensitivity profile
    e. Spatial profile

17. The thickness of the section in CT depends primarily on:
    a. kVp
    b. mAs
    c. Matrix size
    d. Pre-detector collimation
    e. Pre-patient collimation

18. CT mA is modulated to:
    a. Improve image contrast
    b. Minimize beam hardening
    c. Reduce patient dose
    d. Reduce scatter radiation
    e. Reduce x-ray tube loading

19. CT is performed at high kVp principally to:
    a. Improve image contrast
    b. Minimize beam hardening
    c. Reduce patient dose
    d. Reduce scatter radiation
    e. Reduce x-ray tube loading

20. Streak artifacts on a CT image are usually due to:
    a. Beam hardening
    b. Bone/soft tissue interface
    c. Bowel gas
    d. Detector imbalance
    e. Metal clips

Worksheet 21-2
CT Image Characteristics
Image Quality
Quality Control

Computed tomography images are composed of discrete pixel values. A number of methods are available for measuring CT image quality and include: spatial resolution, contrast resolution, noise, linearity, and uniformity.

Spatial resolution for all imaging modalities is determined by pixel size. The smaller the pixel, the better the spatial resolution. CT imaging systems allow reconstruction of images followed by postingprocessing tasks which affect spatial resolution. Spatial resolution is best measured by **spatial frequency** and **modulation transfer function (MTF)**. The **spatial frequency** for CT imaging systems is expressed often as line pairs per centimeter (lp/cm) instead of line pair per millimeter (lp/mm). Modulation Transfer function is the ratio of the image to the object as a function of spatial frequency.

Contrast resolution refers to the ability of the imaging system to reproduce objects such as cysts and tumors that do not vary much from surrounding tissue in their x-ray absorption properties.

EXERCISES

1. A 120 × 120 matrix will consist of how many pixels?
   a. 120
   b. 240
   c. 625
   d. 14,400
   e. 65,536

2. What is the pixel size of an image reconstructed from a 24-cm diameter region of interest in a 320 × 320 matrix?
   a. 0.25 mm
   b. 0.5 mm
   c. 0.75 mm
   d. 1.3 mm
   e. 1.5 mm

3. A CT image is made with a 5-mm slice thickness and a 0.5-mm pixel size. What is the size of the voxel?
   a. 0.75 mm^3
   b. 1.00 mm^3
   c. 1.25 mm^3
   d. 1.5 mm^3
   e. 25 mm^3

4. Which of the following Hounsfield unit (HU) values *most* closely represents the value for blood?
   a. −80 HU
   b. −40 HU
   c. −2 HU
   d. 20 HU
   e. 100 HU

5. A CT imaging system has a limiting resolution of 7 lp/cm. An object of what size can be resolved?
   a. 0.35 mm
   b. 0.5 mm
   c. 0.7 mm
   d. 1.4 mm
   e. 3.5 mm

6. Which of the following is characteristic of a CT image but *not* of a conventional radiograph?
   a. Anatomic structures are superimposed.
   b. Better contrast resolution is obtained.
   c. Better spatial resolution is obtained.
   d. More scatter radiation reaches the image receptor.
   e. Overlying and underlying tissues are blurred.

7. An image matrix contains which of the following?
   a. Algorithms
   b. Equations of information
   c. Picture elements
   d. Silver halide information units
   e. Slice sensitivity 1.00

8. A Hounsfield unit:
   a. Has a value from −100 to +100
   b. Has a value from −500 to +500
   c. Is the numeral value of a pixel
   d. Is the numeral value of anode heat generated
   e. Is the volume of a voxel expressed in cubic millimeter

9. The precise pixel value in HU depends on which of the following?
   a. 32 shades of gray
   b. Light field, x-ray beam coincidence
   c. Pixel size
   d. The x-ray attenuation coefficient
   e. X-ray beam size

10. Spatial resolution refers to which of the following?
    a. The ability to classify large low-contrast objects
    b. The ability to identify small high-contrast objects
    c. The ability to identify tissues of varying composition
    d. The binary number system
    e. The constancy of the imaging system over time

11. When a CT image is described, contrast resolution:
    a. Is limited by the MTF of the system
    b. Is limited by the noise of the system
    c. Is not as good as in conventional radiography
    d. Is the same as spatial resolution
    e. Means that contrast material was injected

12. Partial volume artifacts are more likely with:
    a. Higher kVp
    b. Higher mA
    c. Larger pixel size
    d. Thicker slices
    e. Thinner slices

Exercises 13 through 15 refer to the figure below.

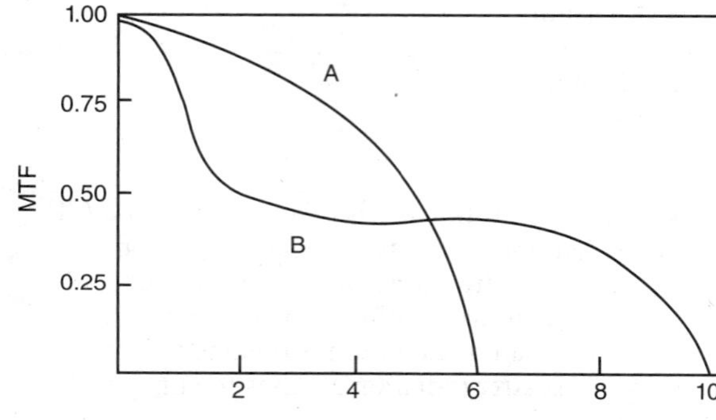

13. The MTF curves describe two imaging systems. Which of the following statements is *true?*
    a. System A detects smaller objects than system B.
    b. System A has better spatial resolution than system B.
    c. System A has more image noise than system B.
    d. System B has better contrast for coarse details than system A.
    e. System B has better spatial resolution than system A.

14. A device has the MTF characteristics represented by B. Which of the following statements is *true* for that device?
    a. At 2 lp/cm, only one-half of an object can be imaged.
    b. At 10 lp/cm, the response is excellent.
    c. It can image a 0.5-mm object.
    d. Its imaging ability increases with increasing spatial frequency.
    e. Longer imaging time than in A will be required.

15. The MTF characteristics of system A suggest that it:
    a. Can image down to approximately 0.8 mm
    b. Can image down to approximately 6 cm
    c. Images large objects better than small objects
    d. Images small objects better than large objects
    e. Is a better system than B

16. Spatial resolution in CT imaging depends principally on:
    a. Focal-spot size
    b. kVp
    c. Pixel size
    d. Post-patient collimation
    e. Slice thickness

Worksheet 21-3 Operational CT Modes

Helical CT reduces motion blur, imaging time, and partial volume artifact. It is made possible by slip-ring technology that allows the gantry to rotate continuously without interruption. Interpolation allows collected data to be reconstructed at any position along the z-axis, which is the long axis of the body. The volume of the tissue image is determined by examination time, couch travel, pitch, and collimation.

The spiral CT pitch is the relationship between patient couch movement and x-ray beam collimation. Increasing the pitch ratio to above 1.0 increases the volume of tissue that can be imaged and reduces patient dose.

Multislice helical CT uses several parallel detector arrays, each of which contains thousands of individual detectors, to produce four or more helical slices at the same time. The signal from each radiation detector is connected to a computer-controlled electronic amplifier and switching device called a *data acquisition system (DAS)*.

The DAS selects detector combinations for signal summation and sends the signals to a computer for image reconstruction. Multislice helical CT can image larger tissue volume faster than single-slice helical CT.

EXERCISES

1. Which of the following terms is equivalent to *helical?*
   a. Elliptical
   b. Spiral
   c. Interpolation
   d. Paraboloid
   e. Trispiral

2. Which of the following molecules takes on a helical structure?
   a. Carbohydrate
   b. Deoxyribonucleic acid
   c. Free radical
   d. Lipid
   e. Protein

3. Which of the following is specifically characteristic of helical CT?
   a. Continuous bidirectional rotation of the x-ray tube
   b. Continuous x-ray tube rotation in one direction
   c. Rotating detector array
   d. Stationary patient couch
   e. Steplike motion of the patient couch

4. During spiral CT examination of a supine patient, the z-axis:
   a. Is the anterior-posterior axis
   b. Is the lateral axis, left to right
   c. Is the lateral axis, right to left
   d. Is the long axis of the body
   e. Varies with the examination

5. The ability to reconstruct an image at any z-axis position is due to:
   a. Extrapolation
   b. Filtered back projection
   c. Fourier transformation
   d. Interpolation
   e. Linear estimation

6. A principal advantage of reconstruction in any z-axis position is:
   a. Image acquisition during a single breath-hold
   b. Improved contrast resolution
   c. Improved spatial resolution
   d. Larger volume of tissue imaged
   e. Reduction of partial volume

7. The simplest form of three-dimensional imaging is:
   a. Isometric
   b. Maximum-intensity projection
   c. Shaded surface display
   d. Shaded volume display
   e. Slip-ring technology

8. Today, all CT scanners are what generation?
   a. First generation
   b. Second generation
   c. Third generation
   d. Fourth generation
   e. Fifth generation

9. During a 360-degree x-ray rotation, the patient couch moves 15 mm during each revolution. Slice thickness is 10 mm. What is the slice pitch?
   a. 0.66
   b. 1.25
   c. 1.5
   d. 1.66
   e. 2.0

10. Which of the following is one advantage of helical CT over conventional CT?
    a. Better patient dose use
    b. Improved contrast resolution
    c. Improved spatial resolution
    d. Lack of motion artifact
    e. Large matrix reconstruction

11. Which of the following is another advantage of helical CT over conventional CT?
    a. Better patient dose use
    b. Improved contrast resolution
    c. Improved spatial resolution
    d. Large matrix reconstruction
    e. Reduced scanning time

12. If a 20-s helical CT examination is acquired at a pitch of 1.5 with collimation of 10 mm, what was the length of the scan if gantry rotation time was 1 s?
    a. 3 cm
    b. 30 cm
    c. 300 cm
    d. 3 mm
    e. 30 mm

13. Thirty centimeters of tissue along the z-axis is to be imaged with a 5-mm slice thickness at a pitch of 2.0. What imaging time is required if gantry rotation time is 1 s?
    a. 20 s
    b. 25 s
    c. 30 s
    d. 35 s
    e. 40 s

14. How much z-axis tissue will be imaged during a 20-s procedure if the slice width is 5 mm at a pitch of 1 and the gantry rotation time is 2 s?
    a. 5 cm
    b. 10 cm
    c. 100 cm
    d. 5 mm
    e. 10 mm

15. Why is it recommended that beam pitch should *not* exceed 2.0?
    a. Increased noise
    b. Poor contrast resolution
    c. Poor patient dose use
    d. Poor spatial resolution
    e. Poor z-axis resolution

16. Which of the following is another term for slice thickness?
    a. Dose profile
    b. Interpolation profile
    c. Reconstruction index
    d. Section sensitivity profile
    e. Z-axis profile

17. With increasing slice pitch:
    a. Image noise is reduced.
    b. Patient dose is increased.
    c. Sagittal/coronal reconstruction is improved.
    d. The section sensitivity profile decreases in width.
    e. The section sensitivity profile increases in width.

18. When a shaded surface display reformation is implemented, the image will appear:
    a. As CT angiography
    b. As z-axis reformation
    c. Isometric
    d. Surface-rendered
    e. Volume-rendered

19. Which of the following technique developments made helical CT possible?
    a. Dose-efficiency detectors
    b. High-frequency generators
    c. Interpolation algorithms
    d. Slip rings
    e. Volume imaging

20. CT angiography relies on a reconstruction process that is called:
    a. Longitudinal reformation
    b. Maximum intensity projection
    c. Shaded surface display
    d. Surface-rendered
    e. Volume-rendered

21. Which of the following characteristics is specific to a helical CT x-ray tube?
    a. High anode heat capacity
    b. High rotation speed
    c. Large effective focal spots
    d. Large target angle
    e. Small effective focal spots

22. Approximately what is the minimum power requirement for the high-voltage generator and x-ray tube for helical CT?
    a. 10 kW
    b. 20 kW
    c. 30 kW
    d. 40 kW
    e. 50 kW

23. The single *most* important advantage of helical CT is which of the following?
    a. Imaging of a large volume of anatomy at a low patient dose
    b. Imaging of a large volume of anatomy in one breath-hold
    c. Improved contrast resolution
    d. Improved spatial resolution
    e. Improved z-axis resolution

24. What range of beam pitch is recommended for multislice spiral CT?
    a. 0.5 to 1
    b. 0.5 to 2
    c. 0.5 to 4
    d. 1
    e. 1 to 2

25. DAS stands for which of the following?
    a. Data acquisition system
    b. Digital acquired space
    c. Digital activation signal
    d. Digital analog server
    e. Digital analog system

26. The largest number of individual detectors in a multislice CT imager is approximately:
    a. Two
    b. Four
    c. Ten
    d. Hundreds
    e. Thousands

27. Which of the following statements about multislice CT is *true?*
    a. Higher-resolution multislice helical CT results in low patient radiation dose.
    b. Larger detector size results in better spatial resolution.
    c. Narrower slice scanning results in better contrast resolution at the same mA.
    d. The simplest approach to multislice scanning is using eight detector arrays, each of equal width.
    e. Wider multislices allow imaging of a greater tissue volume.

28. A principal advantage of multislice helical CT compared with step-and-shoot CT is all of the following *except:*
    a. Better spatial resolution
    b. Faster imaging
    c. Larger tissue volume
    d. Lower patient dose
    e. None of the above

29. Spatial resolution in CT imaging depends principally on:
    a. Focal-spot size
    b. kVp
    c. Pixel size
    d. Postpatient collimation
    e. Slice thickness

30. What was originally the primary disadvantage of third-generation CT scanners?
    a. Long imaging time
    b. Low spatial resolution
    c. Motion artifact
    d. Ring artifact
    e. High heat load

31. What type of material is least likely to produce artifact in a CT image?
    a. High Z-material
    b. Low Z-material
    c. Lead-based material
    d. Aluminum
    e. Copper

32. Which of the following is an advantage of iterative reconstruction methods?
    a. Higher patient dose
    b. Higher spatial resolution
    c. Faster scan time
    d. Higher contrast resolution
    e. Shorter reconstruction time

33. The quantity that describes the ability to distinguish between two different tissues is called:
    a. Contrast resolution
    b. Spatial resolution
    c. Point spread function
    d. Filtered backprojection
    e. Signal-to-noise ratio

34. The standard deviation of a uniform image can help determine:
    a. Spatial resolution
    b. Image noise
    c. Contrast resolution
    d. Patient dose
    e. Scan time

35. What is the primary advantage of a dual-source multislice helical CT?
    a. Lower patient dose
    b. Higher spatial resolution
    c. Less noise
    d. Higher signal-to-noise ratio
    e. Faster scan time

36. What is the HU for water?
    a. 0
    b. 30
    c. −100
    d. 1000
    e. −20

37. A weekly test should be performed to ensure that the Hounsfield unit for water is within what range of its standard value?
    a. ±1
    b. ±5
    c. ±10
    d. ±20
    e. ±100

Worksheet 22-1
Digital Radiographic Tomosynthesis

Tomosynthesis, like so many medical terms, has its roots in Greek. Tomos, in Greek, means slice, a cutting, or a section. Synthesis means a process or the combination of ideas to form a theory or system. The first digital radiographic tomosynthesis (DRT) appeared in digital mammography, as digital breast tomosynthesis (DBT). DBT is now fundamental for screening mammography and diagnostic mammography. DRT is set to replace much of computed tomography (CT) as the imaging modality of choice for many patient conditions.

The main image characteristics of DRT is image contrast.

1. One of the results of replacing CT in the emergency department with DRT is:
   a. Adoption of positioning views
   b. Increased eye lens radiation dose
   c. More precise patient positioning
   d. Not acceptable for orthopedic imaging
   e. Reduced patient radiation dose

2. DRT is a superior image modality compared to digital radiography (DR) in what following characteristic?
   a. Contrast resolution
   b. Noise level
   c. Patient radiation dose
   d. Skeletal imaging
   e. Spatial resolution

3. Which of the following artifacts is unique to DRT?
   a. Backscatter
   b. Blurred-ripple
   c. Ghost
   d. Motion
   e. Pixel drop

4. The association of smaller pixel size with increased patient radiation dose applies to each of the following **except**:
   a. Computed radiography
   b. Computed tomography (CT)
   c. Digital breast tomosynthesis (DBT)
   d. Digital radiography (DR)
   e. Digital radiographic tomosynthesis (DRT)

5. Which of the following correctly describes DRT?
   a. Increased data samples reduce image blur.
   b. Increased data samples increase patient radiation dose.
   c. Increased data samples reduce image noise.
   d. Reduced sweep angle reduces spatial resolution.
   e. Too few data samples can lead to image artifacts

6. What can happen when the sweep angle is increased during DRT?
   a. Improved section resolution
   b. Improved spatial resolution
   c. Reduced patient motion
   d. Reduced patient radiation dose
   e. Reduced section separation

7. Arrange the following medical imaging modalities from least expensive to most expensive for the purchase cost. (1) Computed tomography; (2) diagnostic ultrasound; (3) digital radiographic tomosynthesis; (4) DR; and (5) magnetic resonance imaging
   a. 2, 3, 4, 1, 5
   b. 2, 4, 3, 1, 5
   c. 2, 4, 3, 5, 1
   d. 4, 3, 1, 2, 5
   e. 4, 3, 2, 1, 5

8. Radiographic tomography first appeared in the 1930s. What was its principal contribution to medical imaging?
   a. First digital image modality
   b. Improved image contrast
   c. Improved spatial resolution
   d. Prompted the development of CT
   e. Reduced patient radiation dose

9. What investigation is credited with causing the early acceptance of DRT?
   a. Digital Imaging and Communications in Medicine
   b. Digital Mammography Imaging Study Trial
   c. Mammography Quality Standards Act
   d. Picture Archiving and Communications Systems
   e. Tomosynthesis Mammography Imaging Screening Trial

10. Patient radiation dose following a DRT examination will approximate that following:
    a. DR
    b. Doppler ultrasound
    c. CT
    d. Positron emission tomography (PET)
    e. Single photon emission tomography

11. Which of the following image reconstruction algorithms has **NOT** been applied to DRT?
    a. Algebraic reconstruction
    b. Filtered backprojection
    c. Iterative reconstruction
    d. Maximum likelihood
    e. Quantum reconstruction

12. When performing DRT one should:
    a. Avoid use of patient protective devices
    b. Change pixel size to accommodate the examination goals
    c. Never use a radiographic grid
    d. Obtain many data projections
    e. Occasionally use zero degrees sweep angle

13. What is the major impact due to the number of data projections that are sampled during DRT?
    a. Image quality
    b. Number of images
    c. Patient radiation dose
    d. Section separation
    e. Throughput

14. What are the two methods described for x-ray tube movement during DRT?
    a. Continuous and pause
    b. Continuous and step and shoot
    c. Stagger and continuous
    d. Stagger and pause
    e. Step and shoot and stagger

15. With which medical imaging modality does DRT principally compete?
    a. Computed radiography
    b. CT
    c. DR
    d. Functional magnetic resonance imaging
    e. PET

16. Adoption of DRT is accompanied by what result?
    a. Allows access to computer-aided detection (CAD)
    b. Lowest number of images acquired
    c. Practice as low as reasonably achievable
    d. Reduced image storage requirements
    e. Shortest examination time

17. Which of the following correctly relates DR to DRT to synthesized digital radiography?
    a. A DR can be synthesized from a DRT with additional x-ray exposure.
    b. Reduced patient motion results.
    c. Synthesized DR can produce a computed tomography image from a DRT.
    d. Synthesized DR is possible with the same patient radiation dose as DRT.
    e. The synthesized DR is then called a computed tomography image.

18. What is the meaning of CAD?
    a. Captured answers to diagnosis
    b. Convoluted analog-digital
    c. Convoluted and digital
    d. Computer-aided detection
    e. Computer-aided diagnosis

19. What is one term that can be used to describe tissues imaged using DR?
    a. Extended
    b. Tomosynthesized
    c. Sectioned
    d. Superimposed
    e. Synthesized

20. What is the principal advantage to DRT?
    a. Better spatial resolution
    b. Faster interpretation time
    c. Improved image contrast
    d. Reduced patient radiation dose
    e. Three-dimensional imaging

Worksheet 22-2
Conventional Tomography

Tomography requires deliberate and controlled motion unsharpness. The principal purpose of tomography is to improve image contrast; however, this improvement occurs at the expense of increased patient dose. Tomography was previously utilized with screen-film image receptors and has rapidly disappeared with the development of digital radiographic tomosynthesis (DRT) or simply tomosynthesis.

Tomography involves the joined movement of the x-ray tube and the image receptor to blur issue on either side of the plane of the fulcrum.

1. During conventional tomography, the image receptor:
   a. Is focused on the angle of movement
   b. Is focused on the automatic plane of interest
   c. Moves opposite the x-ray tube in a seesaw motion
   d. Moves with the x-ray tube similarly to the x-ray tube tower assembly in fluoroscopy
   e. Remains fixed

2. During conventional tomography, structures that lie outside the object plane are blurred because of which of the following?
   a. Absorption blur
   b. Geometric blur
   c. Image receptor blur
   d. Motion blur
   e. Subject blur

3. With linear tomography, which of the following is true?
   a. The source and the image receptor are the same distance from the focal plane.
   b. The source and the image receptor cover different tomographic angles.
   c. The source and the image receptor move at the same speed.
   d. The source and the image receptor move in opposite directions.
   e. The source and the image receptor move at the same distance.

4. Which of the following combinations determines the thickness of the cut in a tomograph?
   a. Collimation and filtration
   b. Source-to-image receptor distance (SID) and length of tube travel
   c. Object-to-image receptor distance and speed of tube travel
   d. SID and speed of tube travel
   e. Source-to-object distance and length of tube travel

5. Conventional tomography uses which of the following principles?
   a. Tridimensional image
   b. Optical illusion
   c. Motion blur
   d. Random movement
   e. Stereoscopy

6. During conventional tomography, the fulcrum is in the:
   a. Image plane
   b. Focal plane
   c. Image receptor plane
   d. Object plane
   e. Tomographic layer

7. When the tomographic angle is 0 degrees, the tomographic layer is:
   a. Indefinable
   b. Infinity
   c. Thin
   d. Very thick
   e. Zero

8. To obtain a tomographic layer of approximately 1 mm, the tomographic angle should be approximately:
   a. 10 degrees
   b. 20 degrees
   c. 40 degrees
   d. 50 degrees
   e. 60 degrees

9. Which of the following is the major disadvantage of conventional tomography?
   a. Cost
   b. Enhanced contrast
   c. Image blur
   d. Lost spatial resolution
   e. Patient dose

10. The major advantage of conventional tomography is better:
    a. Contrast resolution
    b. Reproducibility
    c. Image blur
    d. Patient dose
    e. Spatial resolution

11. Conventional tomography has been called which of the following?
    a. Cisternography
    b. Heel effect
    c. Laminography
    d. Myelography
    e. The line-focus principle

12. Which of the following tomographic angles would be considered for use in zonography?
    a. 5 degrees
    b. 15 degrees
    c. 25 degrees
    d. 35 degrees
    e. 60 degrees

13. The tomographic angle is the angle of x-ray tube movement during which of the following?
    a. Anode preparation
    b. Cathode boost
    c. Fulcrum adjustment
    d. Fulcrum motion
    e. X-ray exposure

Worksheet 23-1 Patient Factors

The radiologic technologist has control over the following: exposure technique factors, patient factors, and image quality factors.

Radiographic technique is the selection of the proper x-ray exposure factors with the x-ray imaging system necessary to produce a high-quality radiograph.

The two principal patient factors are the thickness of the body part that is being examined and its composition. In general, the thicker and more dense the part is, the higher the voltage and milliampere-seconds settings should be.

EXERCISES

1. The chest represents high-contrast anatomy (high subject contrast). Therefore which of the following is most appropriate?
   a. High kVp
   b. High mAs
   c. Long source-to-image receptor distance (SID)
   d. Low kVp
   e. Low mAs

2. The anatomic part to be examined must be measured because:
   a. A change of focal spots may be required.
   b. A different image receptor may be required.
   c. The mass density of the part is determined by thickness.
   d. The selected radiographic technique depends on anatomy thickness.
   e. The source-to-skin distance (SSD) changes with anatomy thickness.

3. In general, a chest radiograph should be taken with:
   a. A generalization about this is not possible; decisions are dependent on thickness.
   b. High kVp and high mAs
   c. High kVp and low mAs
   d. Low kVp and high mAs
   e. Low kVp and low mAs

4. What is the effective atomic number of fat?
   a. 6.3
   b. 7.4
   c. 7.6
   d. 10.5
   e. 13.8

5. What is the effective atomic number of lung tissue?
   a. 6.3
   b. 7.4
   c. 7.6
   d. 10.5
   e. 13.8

6. What is the effective atomic number of soft tissue?
   a. 6.3
   b. 7.4
   c. 7.6
   d. 10.5
   e. 13.8

7. What is the effective atomic number of bone?
   a. 6.3
   b. 7.4
   c. 7.6
   d. 10.5
   e. 13.8

8. For a given anatomic part, the smallest change in mAs that can be perceived on the radiographic image is approximately:
   a. 5%
   b. 15%
   c. 30%
   d. 50%
   e. 70%

9. Which of the following tissue characteristics is most important when photoelectric interaction prevails, as in mammography?
   a. Effective atomic number
   b. Electron density
   c. Mass density
   d. Tissue thickness
   e. Tissue shape

10. Which of the following tissue characteristics is most important when Compton interaction prevails, as in computed tomography?
    a. Effective atomic number
    b. Electron density
    c. Mass density
    d. Tissue Thickness
    e. Tissue shape

Worksheet 23-2
Image Quality Factors

Radiographic technique factors set by the radiologic technologist consist of current, exposure time (ms), voltage, and SID (cm). These factors influence the radiographic exposure to the patient. The selected combination of these factors determines the quality of the radiograph. **Image quality factors** refer to terms used to evaluate the characteristics of a radiographic image. The principal terms are **image receptor (IR) response**, **contrast resolution, spatial resolution**, and **distortion**.

The radiologic technologist selects a combination of exposure technique factors to produce a radiograph with an acceptable scale of contrast, spatial and contrast resolution, and minimal distortion of the image.

EXERCISES

1. If a radiographic technique calling for 100 mA at 100 ms is changed to 50 mA at 2000 ms:
   a. Grayscale contrast will become longer.
   b. Grayscale contrast will become shorter.
   c. There will be no change in grayscale contrast.
   d. There will be no change in exposed time.
   e. There will be no change in x-ray tube capacity.

2. A longer grayscale on a radiograph can be obtained by doing which of the following?
   a. Increasing kVp
   b. Increasing mAs
   c. Reducing kVp
   d. Reducing mAs
   e. Using a larger focal spot

3. For a mobile abdominal radiographic examination, radiographic contrast can be increased by doing which of the following?
   a. Increasing the kVp and decreasing the mAs
   b. Increasing the object-to-image receptor distance (OID)
   c. Increasing the SID
   d. Doubling the mAs
   e. Using a high-ratio grid

4. A radiograph that exhibits a long grayscale contrast has which of the following features?
   a. Few shades of gray that have great differences
   b. Few shades of gray that have minimal differences
   c. Good spatial resolution
   d. Many shades of gray that have great differences
   e. Many shades of gray that have minimal differences

5. From the following set of exposure technique factors, select the set that is most likely to produce a radiograph with the best spatial resolution:
   a. A
   b. B
   c. C
   d. D
   e. E

	mAs	kVp	OID	SID	Focal Spot
A	10	60	8 cm	90 cm	2.0 mm
B	20	68	10 cm	90 cm	2.0 mm
C	25	72	5 cm	180 cm	1.0 mm
D	30	86	5 cm	90 cm	1.0 mm
E	50	94	4 cm	100 cm	1.0 mm

6. Which of the preceding exposure technique factors would result in the worst spatial resolution?
   a. A
   b. B
   c. C
   d. D
   e. E

7. If a radiographic technique designed for an 8:1 grid is changed to accommodate a 10:1 grid:
   a. Grayscale contrast will become longer.
   b. Grayscale contrast will become shorter.
   c. There will be no change in contrast resolution.
   d. There will be no change in grayscale contrast.
   e. There will be no change in x-ray tube capacity.

8. Which of the following is the function of optimizing contrast?
   a. To control detail sharpness
   b. To control quantum noise
   c. To increase brightness
   d. To improve spatial resolution
   e. To distinguish between structures of similar densities

9. A radiographic technique that would ensure visibility of detail for a cervical spine is:
   a. Increasing the OID
   b. Reducing the SID
   c. Reducing the SSD
   d. Selecting the large focal spot
   e. Using a beam restriction device

10. A radiograph was made using these factors: 200 mA, 300 ms, 70 kVp, 100 cm SID. A mobile radiograph is then conducted at 80 cm. To maintain exposure to the IR, approximately what mAs should be selected?
    a. 15 mAs
    b. 20 mAs
    c. 28 mAs
    d. 38 mAs
    e. 48 mAs

11. Exercises 11 through 13 refer to the following exposure technique factors:
    a. 100 mA, 500 ms, 60 kVp, no grid
    b. 200 mA, 750 ms, 50 kVp, 16:1 grid
    c. 400 mA, 100 ms, 60 kVp, no grid
    d. 600 mA, 700 ms, 70 kVp, 8:1 grid
    e. 800 mA, 200 ms, 80 kVp, 8:1 grid

12. Which technique factors should result in the greatest latitude?
    a. A
    b. B
    c. C
    d. D
    e. E

13. Which technique factors should result in the highest contrast?
    a. A
    b. B
    c. C
    d. D
    e. E

14. Which technique factors should result in the highest patient dose?
    a. A
    b. B
    c. C
    d. D
    e. E

15. If a technique of 100 mA, 1000 ms is changed to 200 mA, 500 ms:
    a. There will be a reduction in the contrast resolution.
    b. There will be an increase in contrast resolution.
    c. Patient dose will increase.
    d. There will be no change in contrast resolution.
    e. There will be no change in patient dose.

Worksheet 23-3 Distortion

To obtain a high-quality radiograph, an understanding of geometry is necessary. The x-ray source, the anatomic object, and the image receptor all lie in different planes; therefore the image will always be larger than the object—a condition called magnification. Under some circumstances (e.g., cerebral angiography and mammography), magnification is desired and planned. Normally, however, it is preferable to have as little magnification as possible.

The degree of magnification is identified by the magnification factor (MF).

$$MF = \frac{\text{Image size}}{\text{Object size}} = \frac{\text{SID}}{\text{SOD}}$$

The size of the object is rarely accessible for measurement; consequently, the MF usually is determined by the ratio of SID to SOD. SOD usually can be estimated accurately.

Image **distortion** occurs when the object is not positioned in a plane that is parallel to the plane of the image receptor. This situation occurs frequently in clinical practice and is one of the principal reasons why precise patient positioning is necessary.

EXERCISES

1. Image magnification increases with increasing:
   a. Image size
   b. Object size
   c. OID
   d. SID
   e. SOD

2. 2. Distortion primarily occurs:
   a. Because subject anatomy is inclined
   b. Because subject anatomy is thick rather than thin
   c. When improper kVp was selected
   d. When subject anatomy is flat
   e. When subject anatomy lies parallel to the image receptor

3. Distortion:
   a. Can be corrected by proper patient positioning
   b. Is controlled by focal-spot size
   c. Never accompanies magnification
   d. Occurs only lateral to the central axis of the x-ray beam
   e. Occurs only when the image is inclined

4. To reduce magnification, one should do which of the following?
   a. Reduce OID
   b. Reduce SID
   c. Reduce SSD
   d. Use the small focal spot
   e. Use tighter collimation

5. If the SID is 100 cm and an object is placed 20 cm from the image receptor, what is the MF?
   a. 0.8
   b. 1.0
   c. 1.25
   d. 1.4
   e. 1.6

6. In a particular radiographic examination, the SID is 100 cm and the SOD is 86 cm. The image size-to-object size ratio is approximately:
   a. 0.86:1
   b. 1.12:1
   c. 1.16:1
   d. 2.14:1
   e. 3:1

7. Distortion of an x-ray image results from unequal:
   a. Exposure of the object
   b. Focal spot
   c. Heel effect
   d. Magnification
   e. SID

8. In magnification radiography, when the object is placed equidistant between the source and the image receptor, the size of the image will be:
   a. 1.33 times object size
   b. 2.0 times object size
   c. Four times object size
   d. One-half the object size
   e. The same size as the object

9. A 20-cm object is radiographed at 40 cm from the focal spot, and the SID is 60 cm. The size of the image will be:
   a. 30 cm
   b. 40 cm
   c. 50 cm
   d. 60 cm
   e. 70 cm

10. When an object is present on one side of the central axis of the x-ray beam:
    a. Distortion will disappear.
    b. Subject contrast will remain unchanged.
    c. The MF will be larger.
    d. The MF will be smaller.
    e. The MF will remain unchanged.

11. To obtain minimum magnification, one should do which of the following?
    a. Make sure the object is positioned on the central axis.
    b. Position the anatomy close to the image receptor.
    c. Select a short SID.
    d. Select a short SSD.
    e. Use maximum collimation.

12. Which of the following conditions contributes least to image distortion?
    a. A thick object at a short SID
    b. A thin object at a long SID
    c. Angling of the central ray
    d. Object position
    e. Off-axis imaging

13. To minimize magnification, one should do which of the following?
    a. Position the object as close to the image receptor as is practical
    b. Position the x-ray tube as close to the patient as is practical
    c. Use high kVp, low mAs
    d. Use the large focal spot
    e. Use the small focal spot

14. A foreshortened image:
    a. Can be corrected by increasing kVp and reducing mAs
    b. Can be corrected by reducing kVp and increasing mAs
    c. Can be corrected by reducing SID
    d. Can never be smaller than the object
    e. Results from an inclined object

15. Image magnification can be reduced with the use of which of the following?
    a. A cone
    b. Increased filtration
    c. Shorter OID
    d. Shorter SID
    e. Shorter SSD

16. Which of the following is not one of the geometric factors that affect radiographic quality?
    a. Collimation
    b. Distortion
    c. Focal-spot size
    d. Magnification
    e. SID

17. The MF is not dependent on:
    a. Focal-spot size
    b. OID
    c. SOD
    d. SSD
    e. SID

18. The MF increases with increasing:
    a. Focal-spot size
    b. OID
    c. SID
    d. SOD
    e. SSD

Worksheet 23-4
Improving Radiographic Quality

The radiologic technologist has many decisions to make before performing a patient examination, each of which will influence the quality of the resultant radiographic image. These decisions relate to the choice of equipment, patient preparation and positioning, and selection of radiographic factors from the operating console. In general, a change in the selection of one factor will influence the selection of other factors; however, this is not always the case.

EXERCISES

1. Magnification is reduced by which of the following?
   a. Increasing kVp
   b. Decreasing SID and OID
   c. Increasing SID and OID
   d. Increasing SID and reducing OID
   e. Reducing focal-spot size

2. Focal-spot blur can be reduced by which of the following?
   a. Increasing kVp
   b. Increasing mAs
   c. Increasing the OID
   d. Reducing SOD
   e. Using the small focal spot

3. When radiographic technique factors are adjusted to provide an acceptable image and then filtration is added to the x-ray tube, which of the following will increase?
   a. Average energy of the x-ray beam
   b. Image noise
   c. Patient dose
   d. Radiographic contrast
   e. Spatial resolution

4. Use of contrast media principally improves which of the following?
   a. Blur
   b. Contrast resolution
   c. Mass density of the tissue
   d. Image brightness
   e. Spatial Resolution

5. Reducing field size through proper collimation usually results in improved:
   a. Blur
   b. Contrast resolution
   c. Magnification
   d. Patient dose
   e. Spatial resolution

6. Which of the following is most often influenced by focal-spot size?
   a. Absorption blur
   b. Contrast resolution
   c. Geometric blur
   d. Motion blur
   e. Patient dose

7. In a radiographic examination of the lumbar spine, which of the following techniques would result in greatest exposure to the patient?
   a. 70 kVp/200 mAs
   b. 80 kVp/100 mAs
   c. 95 kVp/50 mAs
   d. 110 kVp/25 mAs
   e. 120 kVp/25 mAs

8. Which of the following does not affect image blur?
   a. Focal-spot size
   b. kVp
   c. OID
   d. SID
   e. SOD

9. Which of the following is the principal reason for using direct-exposure radiography?
   a. Better resolution of low-contrast tissues
   b. Better spatial resolution
   c. Higher contrast
   d. Less motion blur
   e. Lower patient dose

10. An anteroposterior examination of the abdomen is taken at 80 kVp, 50 mAs, and 100 cm SID. If the scale of contrast is to be shortened, the radiologic technologist must do which of the following?
    a. Increase both mAs and kVp
    b. Reduce both mAs and kVp
    c. Reduce kVp and increase mAs
    d. Reduce mAs and increase kVp
    e. Shorten the SID

11. Assume that the usual exposure time for a lateral cervical spine radiograph at 100 cm SID is 100 ms. At an SID of 90 cm, all other factors remaining the same, the correct exposure time would be:
    a. 10 ms
    b. 25 ms
    c. 50 ms
    d. 80 ms
    e. 180 ms

12. When radiographic technique factors are adjusted to obtain an acceptable image, patient dose will increase as which of the following increases?
    a. OID
    b. Grid ratio
    c. SID
    d. SOD
    e. SSD

13. Magnification can be reduced by which of the following?
    a. Decreasing SID and increasing OID
    b. Decreasing SSD and increasing SID
    c. Increasing SID and decreasing OID
    d. Increasing SSD and increasing OID
    e. Reducing focal-spot size

14. When technique factors are adjusted to obtain an acceptable image, motion blur will increase with which of the following?
    a. Increase in focal-spot size
    b. Increased field size
    c. Low-ratio grid (compared with high-ratio grid)
    d. Increased total filtration
    e. Increased length of exposure

Worksheet 24-1 Photometric Quantities

The adoption of digital imaging brings with it a new set of required physics skills. In addition to the physics of ionizing radiation, we must have an understanding of the physics of visible light and how it affects image interpretation. Photometry is the science of visible light, including its emission, reflection, and measurement. The basic unit of photometry is the lumen, which quantifies the intensity of light from a source.

A major advantage of digital imaging is that it allows one to preprocess and postprocess the image to accentuate image detail. Further, the digital image can be viewed by different people in different locations through the picture archiving and communication system (PACS).

EXERCISES

1. Photometry is the science of the:
   a. Anatomy of human vision
   b. Measurement of photographic images
   c. Quantity of light
   d. Reflection and refraction of light
   e. Measurement of the response of the human eye to light

2. The postprocessing manipulation called *image inversion* refers to:
   a. Changing from landscape to portrait format
   b. Exchange of images
   c. Reorienting right and left
   d. Reorienting top and bottom
   e. Turning white-black to black-white

3. Photopic vision is associated with:
   a. Night vision
   b. Cone vision
   c. Dim light
   d. Black and white vision
   e. Rod vision

4. How does one preprocess a digital image to correct for pixel, row, or column defects?
   a. Dark reference correction
   b. Extrapolation algorithms
   c. Interpolation algorithms
   d. Offset correction
   e. Pixel reregistration

5. Which of the following describes the luminous intensity from a light source such as a lightbulb?
   a. Cosine law
   b. Illuminance
   c. Luminance
   d. Luminance intensity
   e. Luminous flux

6. What is the approximate illuminance of an indoor tennis court?
   a. 5 fc
   b. 20 fc
   c. 30 fc
   d. 100 fc
   e. 200 fc

7. The luminance of a digital display device is measured in:
   a. Candelas
   b. Candelas per meter squared
   c. Foot-candles
   d. Lumens
   e. Luxes

8. What is the matrix array of a 5-megapixel digital display device?
   a. 500 × 1000 pixels
   b. 1000 × 1000 pixels
   c. 1200 × 1800 pixels
   d. 1500 × 2000 pixels
   e. 2000 × 2500 pixels

9. Which of the following is characteristic of a cathode ray tube (CRT) but not of an active-matrix liquid-crystal display (AMLCD)?
   a. Active matrix address
   b. Flat face
   c. Light modulating
   d. Square pixel
   e. Veiling glare

10. What unit is used to describe illuminance, the intensity of light incident on a surface?
    a. Candela
    b. Candela per meter squared
    c. Foot-candle
    d. Lumen
    e. Nit

11. The luminance of a mammography viewbox must be uniform and at least 3000 nits. What is a nit?
    a. Candela per foot squared
    b. Candela per meter squared
    c. Lumen per foot squared
    d. Lumen per meter squared
    e. Lumen per steradian

12. With digital radiography, the cosine law applies to:
    a. Grayscale imaging
    b. Image inversion
    c. Inverse square law
    d. Off-axis viewing
    e. Reduced spatial resolution

13. Compared with photopic vision, scotopic vision:
    a. Has better spatial resolution
    b. Involves cones
    c. Is bright light vision
    d. Is more color vision
    e. Occurs at shorter wavelengths

14. An active matrix liquid crystal display is better than a cathode-ray tube display because:
    a. Of its light-emitting property.
    b. Of its phosphor face.
    c. It has a curved face.
    d. It is a light-modulating device.
    e. It uses a scanning electron beam.

15. Liquid crystals are:
    a. Linear organic molecules
    b. Phosphor grains
    c. Photo detecting devices
    d. Thin film transistors
    e. Solid grains embedded in glass

16. The aperture ratio refers to the:
    a. Ability to control individual pixels
    b. Percent of light transmission
    c. Size of a pixel
    d. Size of the liquid crystals
    e. Viewing of an image off-axis

17. Ergonomics is the study of:
    a. Hospital information systems
    b. Human factors applied to system design
    c. Light levels in work areas
    d. Light illumination of workstations
    e. PACSs

18. All of the following are examples of image preprocessing *except*:
    a. Window and level
    b. Offset correction
    c. Flatfielding
    d. Gain correction
    e. Signal interpolation

19. Which of the following postprocessing methods helps improve visualization and spatial resolution?
    a. Annotation
    b. Magnification
    c. Image flip
    d. Image inversion
    e. Edge enhancement

20. PACS' primary use is to:
    a. Postprocess an image
    b. Preprocess an image
    c. Store digital images
    d. Invert an image
    e. Increase the size of the file room

Worksheet 25-1
Electronic Programs

Of all the members of the medical imaging team, the radiologist is ultimately responsible for the interpretation of medical images, but every member of the team, particularly the radiologic technologist (RT), has responsibilities. Radiologists and RTs interact most directly with picture archiving and communication systems (PACS) and radiology information systems (RIS). The RIS deals with schedules, protocol descriptors, diagnostic conclusions, and billing. PACS deals strictly with image manipulation and document storage.

1. Which of the following electronic medical imaging programs was introduced first?
   a. Computer-aided detection/diagnosis
   b. Digital Imaging and Communication in Medicine (DICOM)
   c. Health Level 7 (HL7)
   d. ACS
   e. RIS

2. The four principal components of a PACS include each of the following except the:
   a. Acquisition system
   b. Display system
   c. Network
   d. Storage system
   e. Workstation

3. A client of a medical imaging network would include each of the following except:
   a. An imaging system
   b. HIS (hospital information system)
   c. Mainframe computer
   d. RIS
   e. Satellite clinic

4. The purpose of DICOM is to:
   a. Develop ontologies
   b. Identify the best workflow
   c. Present metadata
   d. Process textual data
   e. Produce images in a standard format

5. Pre-fetching in electronic medical imaging refers to:
   a. Coding of disease
   b. Coding of radiologic procedures
   c. Implementing image integration profiles
   d. Recalling archived images
   e. Storing archived images

6. Which is one of the main responsibilities of the RT regarding electronic image handling?
   a. Approve IHE (Integrating the Healthcare Enterprise) integration with imaging modality.
   b. Making structured reports easily searchable
   c. Input and check of header metadata
   d. Ensure that the DICOM vendor is compliance approved
   e. Transfer of images to radiologist

7. When one Googles a word or phrase, a list of answers appears. Who would prepare that list and the order of appearance?
   a. A bonder
   b. A coder
   c. A lister
   d. The RIS (Radiology Information System) team
   e. The IT (Information Technology) team.

8. RadLex would most likely be used by the
   a. Administrator.
   b. Medical physicist.
   c. Radiologic technologist.
   d. Radiologist.
   e. Service engineer.

9. Which of the following electronic medical imaging programs support digital image acquisition, interpretation, and storage?
   a. HIS
   b. HL7
   c. IHE
   d. PACS
   e. RIS

10. *Network* in medical imaging refers to
    a. Commands for transfer, use, and storage of images
    b. Imaging modalities
    c. Image modality worklist
    d. The interaction of many computers
    e. Medical specialties outside of radiology

11. Which of the following exploded in frequency of application during COVID-19?
    a. Computed tomography (CT)
    b. Nuclear medicine
    c. PACS
    d. RIS
    e. Teleradiology

12. A CT examination results in 60 images, each with matrix size 512 × 512 and 256 shades of gray. Approximately how much digital storage is required?
    a. 1.0 MB
    b. 1.5 MB
    c. 2.0 MB
    d. 4.0 MB
    e. 10.0 MB

13. The properties *lexicon* and *ontology* refer to:
    a. Media storage standards
    b. Security management profiles
    c. Standardized terms and vocabulary
    d. The electronic definition of objects
    e. World-Wide Web services for DICOM devices

14. The Common Procedural Terminology (CPT) codes now number in excess of ____ different medical conditions for patients.
    a. 1000
    b. 5000
    c. 10,000
    d. 15,000
    e. 50,000

15. Which of the following electronic medical imaging programs supports patient scheduling and digital image protocols?
    a. HIS
    b. HL7
    c. IHE
    d. PACS
    e. RIS

16. Which of the following best describes Teleradiology?
    a. Commands for image transfer, use, and storage
    b. Image display standards
    c. Requirements for DICOM compliance
    d. Remote transmission for digital image viewing
    e. Sending textual information between systems

17. What is the information management and database part of PACS?
    a. DICOM
    b. HL7
    c. Image modality
    d. Image modality worklist
    e. RIS

18. BI-RADS is the acronym for
    a. Back Injury—Relaxed and Distressed Symptoms
    b. Back Involved with Recall and Discharge Service
    c. Bone Irregularity—Recent and Distant Signs
    d. Breast Imaging Reporting and Data Systems
    e. Breast Irregularity Registered and Diagnosed Specialty

19. PACS includes all of the following *except:*
    a. DICOM
    b. EMR (electronic medical record)
    c. HIS
    d. RIS
    e. Protocol worklist

20. Which electronic medical imaging program is most helpful to the radiologist with image read, viewing, and interpretation?
    a. EMR
    b. HIS
    c. IHE
    d. PACS
    e. RIS

21. The principal application of DICOM is to:
    a. Describe symptoms and disease
    b. Describe the medical imaging procedure
    c. Process medical images
    d. Process textual data
    e. Process workflow profiles

Worksheet 26-1 Digital Display Device Performance Assessment

Assessing the performance of digital display devices requires that we have some understanding of the field of photometry. Numerous initiatives have been developed to standardize soft copy digital display device performance standards.

1. Digital image spatial resolution is determined by
   a. AAPM TG 18-CX pattern
   b. AAPM TG 18-QC pattern
   c. Contrast resolution
   d. Dynamic range
   e. Pixel size

2. For the assessment of angular dependence when viewing a digital display device, which of the following American Association of Physicists in Medicine (AAPM) TG 18 patterns is used?
   a. Dot size
   b. Half moons
   c. Line-pair pattern
   d. Square test pattern
   e. Star patterns

3. How can one evaluate ambient light reflected from the screen of a digital display device?
   a. Cycle the room lighting on and off
   b. Turn off the screen
   c. Turn off the screen and room lighting
   d. Turn off the room lighting and cycle the screen on and off
   e. Turn off the room lighting while viewing the screen

4. What instrument should be used to ensure proper ambient light level in a reading room?
   a. Illuminescence meter
   b. Luminance gauge
   c. Luminance meter
   d. Optic meter
   e. Optic range meter

5. Which of the following areas would have an illuminance closest to 2000 lux?
   a. Cloudy day
   b. Full moon
   c. Reading room
   d. Tennis court
   e. Waiting room

6. What is the purpose of the Gray Scale Display Function (GSDF)?
   a. Add balance to Digital Imaging and Communications in Medicine
   b. Define dynamic range
   c. Ensure contrast resolution on any digital display device
   d. Maintain perceived brightness on any digital display device
   e. Organize perceived linearization

7. During the 20th century, image quality control (QC) concentrated on wet chemistry and view boxes. Today, QC concentrates on
   a. Digital display devices and ergonomics
   b. Dry chemistry and wet chemistry
   c. Pixel size and dynamic range
   d. Spatial resolution and contrast resolution
   e. Workstations and reading rooms

8. Digital display device noise principally affects what image characteristic?
   a. Artifacts
   b. Contrast resolution
   c. Dynamic range
   d. Pixel size
   e. Spatial resolution

9. Maximum nonuniformity for an individual digital display device should be less than what value?
   a. 5%
   b. 10%
   c. 20%
   d. 30%
   e. 50%

10. The evaluation of luminance nonuniformity
    a. Is a qualitative assessment
    b. Is a quantitative assessment
    c. Is a visual assessment
    d. Requires measurement of L_{max} and L_{min}
    e. Requires measurement of *P* values

11. Which of the following image distortions is **not** associated with a digital display device?
    a. Distance
    b. Object shape
    c. Pincushion
    d. Pixel deletion
    e. Size

12. Which of the following areas would have an illumination closest to 10 lux?
    a. Cloudy day
    b. Hallway
    c. Reading room
    d. Tennis court
    e. Waiting room

13. What organization produced the electronic test pattern identified as the SMPTE pattern?
    a. Social Management of Personnel Trained and Excellent
    b. Society of Major Pathology and Teleradiology Engineers
    c. Society of Managers of Photographic Technique and Excellence
    d. Society of Motion Picture and Television Engineers
    e. Society of Movers in Principal Task Experience

14. QC monitoring of a digital display device is principally the responsibility of which team member?
    a. Department director
    b. Medical physicist
    c. Radiologic technologist
    d. Radiologist
    e. Service engineer

15. Percent nonuniformity is calculated with the use of which of the following?
    a. $100(L_{max}+L_{min})/(L_{max}-L_{min})$
    b. $100(L_{max}+L_{min})(L_{max}-L_{min})$
    c. $100(L_{max}-L_{min})/(L_{max}+L_{min})$
    d. $100(L_{max}+L_{min})$
    e. $100(L_{max}-L_{min})$

16. Best viewing of an image on a digital display device is
    a. Determined by $L_{max} - L_{min}$
    b. Determined by *P* value range
    c. Straight on
    d. Within $+/-10°$
    e. Within $+/-30°$

17. What is the difference between specular reflection and diffuse reflection from a digital display device?
    a. Luminous reflection versus illuminance reflection
    b. Mirror-like reflection versus cloudy reflection
    c. No distortion reflection versus distortion reflection
    d. Noiseless reflection versus noisy reflection
    e. Pincushion reflection versus barrel reflection

18. What instrument is used to perform QC luminescence measurements of digital display devices?
    a. Dosimeter
    b. Luminous gauge
    c. Luminometer
    d. Photometer
    e. Tonometer

19. Which of the following standard procedures should be applied by the QC technologist regularly to each digital display device?
    a. AAPM TG 18
    b. DIN 2001
    c. GSDF
    d. SMPTE
    e. VESA

20. For which of the following is the SMPTE pattern usually employed?
    a. Artifacts
    b. Contrast resolution
    c. Luminance
    d. Noise
    e. Spatial resolution

21. With regard to a digital display device, what is the difference between luminescence and illuminescence?
    a. Luminescence is light emitted; illuminescence is incident light
    b. Luminescence is measured in l/m^2; illuminescence is measured in cd/m^2
    c. Luminescence relates to a workstation; illuminescence relates to teleradiology
    d. Luminescence relates to individual monitors; illuminescence relates to a bank of monitors
    e. Luminescence relates to stationary imaging; illuminescence relates to the Rolloscope

Worksheet 26-2
Digital Display Quality Control

Quality control activities associated with digital imaging are associated with image receptor response and digital display devices used for image interpretation. Digital display devices may have a number of deficiencies that can interfere with image interpretation. Several organizations have developed electronic test patterns to assess the image quality of a digital display device.

The American Association of Physicists in Medicine (AAPM) has taken the lead in developing electronic test patterns for quality control procedures for digital display devices. These test patterns are designed to be used regularly to evaluate characteristics of digital monitors such as geometric distortion, reflection, resolution, noise, and other features. Users should now use these test patterns in an ordered program of quality control.

EXERCISES

1. Which of the following organizations never developed electronic test patterns for digital display quality control?
   a. ANSI
   b. AAPM
   c. NEMA
   d. SMPTE
   e. VESA

2. 2. GSDF stands for:
   a. Grand source of detected features
   b. Grayscale display function
   c. Great seal of dynamic function
   d. Gross scale of dynamic factors
   e. Ground source determined factor

3. Luminance response of a digital display device is properly accomplished with a/an:
   a. Charge-coupled device
   b. Densitometer
   c. Illuminator
   d. Photometer
   e. Sensitometer

4. This is the AAPM TG-18 QC test pattern. What is it used to evaluate?
   a. Artifacts
   b. Contrast resolution
   c. Geometric distortion
   d. Noise
   e. Spatial resolution

5. This is the AAPM TG-18 AD test pattern. What is it used to evaluate?
   a. Artifacts
   b. Contrast resolution
   c. Diffuse reflection
   d. Geometric distortion
   e. Noise

6. Geometric distortion causes:
   a. Poor overall image visibility
   b. A displayed image to differ in size from the original
   c. Mirror images of surrounding objects
   d. Difficulty in seeing dark objects
   e. Difficulty in seeing small objects

7. Too much noise in an image causes:
   a. Poor overall image visibility
   b. A displayed image to differ in size from the original
   c. Mirror images of surrounding objects
   d. Difficulty in seeing dark objects
   e. Difficulty in seeing small objects

8. This is the AAPM TG-18 CT test pattern, which contains 16 shades of gray. What is it used to evaluate?
   a. Contrast resolution
   b. Diffuse reflection
   c. Geometric distortion
   d. Luminance response
   e. Noise

9. Poor luminance response often results in:
   a. Poor overall image visibility
   b. Displayed image differing in size from the original
   c. Mirror images of surrounding objects
   d. Difficulty in seeing dark objects
   e. Difficulty in seeing small objects

10. Poor display spatial resolution results in:
    a. Poor overall image visibility
    b. Displayed image differing in size from the original
    c. Mirror images of surrounding objects
    d. Difficulty in seeing dark objects
    e. Difficulty in seeing small objects

11. This is the AAPM TG-18 LN test pattern, which contains three images. What is it used to evaluate?
    a. Artifacts
    b. Contrast resolution
    c. Diffuse reflection
    d. Luminance uniformity
    e. Luminance response

12. This is the AAPM TG-18 UN test pattern, which contains three nine-section images. What is it used to evaluate?
    a. Contrast resolution
    b. Diffuse reflection
    c. Geometric distortion
    d. Luminance uniformity
    e. Luminance response

13. This is the AAPM TG-18 CX test pattern. What is it used to evaluate?
    a. Artifacts
    b. Contrast resolution
    c. Geometric distortion
    d. Nonuniformity
    e. Spatial resolution

14. Specular reflection can result in:
    a. Poor overall image visibility
    b. Displayed image differing in size from the original
    c. Mirror images of surrounding objects
    d. Difficulty in seeing dark objects
    e. Difficulty in seeing small objects

15. Images from a digital modality store pixel information as an array of pixels with each pixel containing a:
    a. Digital driving level
    b. Luminance level
    c. Presentation value
    d. Brightness value
    e. Contrast value

16. This is the AAPM TG-18 PX test pattern, which has a rather uniform intensity. What is it used to evaluate?
    a. Contrast resolution
    b. Diffuse reflection
    c. Noise
    d. Nonuniformity
    e. Resolution uniformity

17. This is the AAPM TG-18 AFC test pattern, which contains low-contrast squares. What is it used to evaluate?
    a. Artifacts
    b. Contrast resolution
    c. Luminance
    d. Noise
    e. Nonuniformity

Worksheet 27-1 Computer Applications

Computer applications continue to expand and evolve in medical imaging. The first large-scale radiology application was computed tomography back in the 1970s. Computers control high-voltage x-ray generators and radiographic control panels, making digital fluoroscopy and digital radiography now routine.

Telecommunication systems have provided for the development of teleradiology, which is the transfer of digital images and patient data to remote locations for interpretation. Future applications of **artificial intelligence** and **quantum computing** will extend the value of imaging science in all areas of healthcare in the future.

A computer has two principal parts—hardware and software. The **hardware** is everything about the computer that is visible. Operations include input processing, memory, storage, output, and communications. The **software** consists of computer programs that tell the hardware what to do and how to store and manipulate data.

EXERCISES

1. The principal component of the computer controls the storage and manipulation of data.
   a. Hardware
   b. Software
   c. Hard drive
   d. Processor
   e. Circuit

2. In the 17th century, two mathematicians, Blaise Pascal and Gottfried Leibniz, built mechanical calculators to perform basic arithmetic functions using:
   a. Tabulation machine
   b. Encrypted military codes
   c. Pegged wheels
   d. Electronic digital computer
   e. Abacus

3. The first general-purpose electronic computer was developed in 1946 by:
   a. J. Presper Eckert and John Mauchly
   b. John Atansoff and Clifford Berry
   c. Charles Babbage
   d. Herman Hollerith
   e. William Shockley

4. In 1948 this alternating electronic switch was invented, which directed the flow of electrons in a circuit. This electronic switch is known as the:
   a. Alternator
   b. Battery
   c. Light bulb
   d. Transistor
   e. Generator

5. All computer languages translate the data provided by the user into:
   a. A series of Xs and Os
   b. A series of 1 s and 0 s
   c. Alphabetical order
   d. The periodic table
   e. Alphanumeric order

6. The word, "digit" comes from the Latin word for:
   a. Knee
   b. Eye
   c. Ball
   d. Finger
   e. Carrot

7. Computers utilize a _______ system as their form of communication.
   a. Duodecimal
   b. Octal
   c. Hexadecimal
   d. Tri numeral
   e. Binary

8. Digital images are made of __________ which are arranged in a _______.
   a. Pixels; matrix
   b. Matrix; pixels
   c. Pixels; layers
   d. Volume elements; rows and columns

9. A single binary digit is called:
   a. Bite
   b. Byte
   c. Word
   d. Bit
   e. Sentence

10. Which of the following matrix sizes are used for digital radiography?
    a. 256 × 256
    b. 1024 × 1024
    c. 1024 × 2048
    d. 2048 × 2048
    e. 2048 × 4096

11. If a computer has one (1) gigabyte of memory, how many bytes are represented?
    a. 1000
    b. 10,000
    c. 100,000
    d. 1,000,000
    e. 1,000,000,000

12. A series of instructions, such as "delete file," organizes data through the computer to solve a problem and is provided by the:
    a. Operating system
    b. Software system
    c. Application programs
    d. Software applications
    e. Computer program

13. A computer program that translates computer language such as Java or C++ into machine language the computer can understand is called:
    a. Assembler
    b. Compiler
    c. Processor
    d. Developer
    e. Creator

14. Application programs are also known as "apps" and include the following programs **except:**
    a. Word
    b. PowerPoint
    c. Google Drive
    d. Java
    e. iTunes

15. Which program language was developed as a combination of high-level languages with the functionality of low-level languages and is considered the first modern "programmer's language?"
    a. FORTRAN
    b. Pascal
    c. C
    d. BASIC
    e. COBOL

16. Which program language is used to format pages on the Internet?
    a. JAVA
    b. LOGO
    c. ADA
    d. HTML
    e. CPU

17. Active computer storage is referred to as which of the following:
    a. External memory
    b. Random access memory (RAM)
    c. Secondary memory
    d. Cloud storage
    e. Read-only memory (ROM)

18. Instructions provided by the computer's manufacturer are inertly built into the computer and engaged when the unit is turned on and stored in the:
    a. ROM
    b. RAM
    c. Primary memory
    d. Internal memory
    e. Active storage

19. Flash drives are used as an option for what type of memory storage?
    a. Primary memory
    b. Secondary memory
    c. Internal memory
    d. Cloud memory storage
    e. ROM

20. A byte is a group of how many bits?
    a. 2
    b. 4
    c. 5
    d. 6
    e. 8

21. Higher-capacity hard drives are often measured in which of the following units?
    a. Terabytes
    b. Gigabytes
    c. Megabytes
    d. Kilobytes
    e. Terabits

22. All the following are input/output devices **except:**
    a. Printer
    b. File
    c. Terminal
    d. Liquid crystal display
    e. Light-emitting diode

Worksheet 27-2 Computer Applications within Radiology

Radiologic science continues to expand and extend computer applications along many avenues. Each contributes to the increasing speed, accuracy, and performance of digital imaging to improvements in human healthcare.

Teleradiology is a form of telecommunications and involves the transfer of medical images and patient data. Advances in technology have allowed for the development of faster and faster teleradiology devices and ultimately improved patient care.

EXERCISES

1. The speed or rate data moves across a communications channel is measured in:
   a. Bits per second
   b. Kilobits per second
   c. Megabits per second
   d. Bps
   e. **All choices**

2. High-speed Internet access is identified as:
   a. Basic modem
   b. Dial-up access
   c. **Broadband**
   d. Quick access
   e. Phone line accessible

3. The purpose of teleradiology is to:
   a. **Transfer images to remote sites**
   b. Allow digital image access for onsite radiologists
   c. Transfer physical copies of images to remote sites
   d. Store pictures for archival and retrieval
   e. Live stream of fluoroscopy studies

4. The keyboard and mouse are what type of entry devices?
   a. Output
   b. **Input**
   c. Transitional
   d. Analog
   e. Processor

5. A geometrical pattern that was developed to be machine-readable in the 1950s is now being replaced by the:
   a. Barcode
   b. Scanner
   c. Bitcoin
   d. **QR Code**
   e. Fax machine

6. Radiologists rely on this system to record their dictation in digital format:
   a. Speech Recognition System
   b. Visual Input System
   c. Source Data System
   d. NEMA
   e. **Voice-Recognition System**

7. The US Food and Drug Administration approved the first application allowing mobile phones to be used to view medical images in:
   a. 2010
   b. 2012
   c. 2020
   d. **2022**
   e. 2024

8. Which system has allowed digital image viewing, interpreting, and reporting from anywhere possible?
   a. RIS
   b. **PACS**
   c. HIS
   d. Canon
   e. Hewlett-Packard

Worksheet 28-1 Artificial Intelligence

Artificial Intelligence (AI) functions are in virtually every element of digital imaging today. **AI** is a computer science that deals with the interpretation of radiologic images by simulating human intelligence. While device manufacturers provide excellent training materials, it will often be up to the technologist to describe to a patient what is happening. AI is the adaptation of computer technology to mimic the human mind in cognitive activities such as learning and problem solving.

With the rapid introduction of AI into radiologic imaging, there are many old and new English words applied to AI. An **algorithm** is a step-by-step mathematical instruction used to solve a problem. Machine learning (ML) and deep learning (DL) are AI functions important to medical imaging. **Machine learning** uses AI algorithms to teach the computer to recognize data patterns. **Deep learning** has similar functions as ML. The "deep" in DL refers to the number of hidden algorithmic layers used to analyze the input data.

EXERCISES

1. Other terms for artificial intelligence:
   a. Augmented intelligence
   b. Alternative intelligence
   c. Autonomous intelligence
   d. Arbitrary intellectual
   e. Artificial intellectual

2. Artificial intelligence is defined as:
   a. Human-made computer software mimicking alternative technology
   b. An application that functions as a simulation of human intelligence
   c. An unnecessary tool in the field of radiology
   d. Computer-based training software for humans
   e. A data storage system

3. The first Large Language Model (LLM) was developed by which company?
   a. IBM
   b. NLP
   c. Microsoft
   d. OpenAI
   e. Apple

4. ML involves all of the following except:
   a. Programmer provides data sets and identifies normal and abnormal information for the machine to analyze.
   b. Machine is taught to learn with large collections of data.
   c. Data sets are provided without identifying abnormalities for the machine to determine abnormalities on its own.
   d. ML can be supervised or unsupervised learning.
   e. Machine provides the data sets to the programmer for identifying abnormalities.

5. For the implementation of ML in radiologic imaging, a machine would be trained with data sets comprised of:
   a. Digital images
   b. Medical record numbers
   c. ICD billing codes
   d. Previously dictated reports
   e. Mp4s

6. The "deep" in DL refers to the:
   a. Multiple layers of the LLM
   b. Number of hidden layers of algorithms
   c. Layers of data mining
   d. Programmer's ability to dive deeper into data
   e. Digital module which performs calculations

7. Which of the following government agencies oversee radiology equipment:
   a. NASA
   b. HUD
   c. FTC
   d. USFDA
   e. USAF

8. Vectors enable which of the following processes:
   a. Provide a universal format of data to use between different AI models
   b. Separating data to identify boundaries of a mass
   c. Storage of data
   d. Diagnose a patient
   e. Allows communication between providers

9. An array of numbers is a:
   a. Vector
   b. Digital image
   c. Data set
   d. Network
   e. Bot

10. Image interpretation is traditionally the responsibility of the:
    a. Radiologic technologist
    b. Registered nurse
    c. Radiologist
    d. PA
    e. Provider

11. In radiology, AI can assist with the following processes:
    a. Image interpretation
    b. Generate reports
    c. Image processing
    d. Image analysis
    e. All of the above

12. Data mining can be used with all of the following except:
    a. Improve the quality of radiologic images
    b. Gain access to the patient's billing records
    c. Reduce patient radiation dose
    d. Improve quality control
    e. Discover incidentalomas

13. The US Food and Drug Administration has approved over ______ AI algorithms for radiology applications.
    a. 50
    b. 100
    c. 500
    d. 700
    e. 1000

14. Organizations offering storage capabilities across the network are identified as being:
    a. Cloud-based
    b. Storm-based
    c. Weather-based
    d. Data-mined
    e. Decision-treed

15. The experimental or theoretical measurements of uncertainty are termed:
    a. Meteorology
    b. Microbiology
    c. Metrology
    d. Microeconomics
    e. Metropolis

16. A layered set of networks through which data is processed is known as a:
    a. Neural network
    b. LLM
    c. Predictive algorithm
    d. Cluster
    e. Decision tree

17. The set of digital images included in supervised training includes the:
    a. Known abnormality
    b. Location of the abnormality
    c. Appearance of the abnormality
    d. All of the answers
    e. None of the answers

18. Unsupervised training has the ability to discover previously unknown patterns leading to diagnosis and is a form of:
    a. Clustering
    b. Metrology
    c. Data mining
    d. Data storage
    e. Cloud-based computing

19. The use of AL in medical imaging will improve which of the following:
    a. Cost of equipment
    b. Accuracy
    c. Communication between insurance and provider
    d. Technologist's salary
    e. Billing procedures

20. Digital imaging workflow includes all of the following *except*:
    a. Scheduling the appointment
    b. Image acquisition
    c. Image processing
    d. Image manipulation
    e. Follow up

21. __________ is the final step in the digital imaging workflow that ensures the diagnostic interpretation is received by the referring provider.
    a. Image processing
    b. Image manipulation
    c. Follow up
    d. Image acquisition
    e. Image interpretation

22. Artificial intelligence algorithms currently in the clinical environment are used to speed image interpretation by identifying a region of interest (ROI) for the radiologist's concentration.
    a. Value of interest (VOI)
    b. LUT (Look Up Table)
    c. FOV (Field of View)
    d. ROI
    e. WL (Window Level)

23. Computer-aided diagnosis (CADx) was developed in the 21st century and eventually evolved to computer-aided detection and is represented as:
    a. CADt
    b. CADc
    c. CADd
    d. CADe
    e. CADde

24. If the data sets provided to the AI algorithms do not include features of race, age, gender, sexual orientation, and so on, there may be a concern with which type of bias?
    a. Algorithmic bias
    b. Representativeness bias
    c. Cognitive bias
    d. Implicit bias
    e. Confirmation bias

Worksheet 29-1 Evolution from Classical Physics to Quantum Mechanics

Classical physics was developed in 1687 by Sir Isaac Newton. For approximately 200 years, classical physics described everything that happened in the ordinary everyday world. In the early 1900s, scientists believed that these rules did not work for systems at extreme scales, large or small. In the early 1900s, two groups of scientists began developing formal mathematical descriptions of how the universe works at these extreme scales.

One group developed a comprehensive mathematical description of how forces and particles interact at the extremely small scale of atoms and is now referred to as **Quantum Mechanics**. The mathematics of quantum mechanics describes in precise detail how atoms, elementary particles, and the fundamental forces of nature, except gravity, interact. The second group of scientists developed a concise explanation of the force of gravity and the relationship between matter and energy and is referred to as **General Relativity**.

In the future, **quantum computers** are expected to be exponentially faster in performance and larger in big data management. The speed of quantum computers is expected to be a distinguishing characteristic of availability. Quantum computers operate with the **qubit**, whereas digital computers utilize the bit.

EXERCISES

1. This scientist is credited for describing modern physics in 1687:
   a. Albert Einstein
   b. Wilhelm Roentgen
   c. Sir Isaac Newton
   d. Neils Bohr
   e. Marie Curie

2. Modern physics is also called:
   a. Classical physics
   b. Quantum mechanics
   c. General Relativity
   d. Gravity
   e. Quantum tunneling

3. What year did Wilhelm Roentgen discover x-rays?
   a. 1687
   b. 1795
   c. 1895
   d. 1904
   e. 1917

4. Which scientific explanation describes the force of gravity and the relationship between matter and energy?
   a. Classical Physics
   b. Modern Physics
   c. Quantum Mechanics
   d. General Relativity
   e. Wave-Particle Duality

5. Which scientific explanation and mathematics describes how atoms, elementary particles and the fundamental forces of nature interact, excluding gravity?
   a. Classical Physics
   b. Modern Physics
   c. Quantum Mechanics
   d. General Relativity
   e. Wave-Particle Duality

6. Newton's laws were limited in their ability to describe the effect of gravity on:
   a. Large distance scales
   b. Short distance scales
   c. Earth
   d. Atoms
   e. Nuclear energy

7. Physicists came together in Brussels in 1927 to discuss the mathematics of quantum mechanics at:
   a. Oxford University
   b. The Nobel Committee Conference
   c. Physicists United Conference
   d. The Solvay Conference
   e. Quantum College

8. Which scientist won the Nobel Prize in physics in 1921 for his description of the photoelectric effect?
   a. Neils Bohr
   b. Sir Isaac Newton
   c. Max Born
   d. Erwin Schrodinger
   e. Albert Einstein

9. The Wave-Particle duality phenomena, originally described by Max Planck, describes the inherent wave-like movements and parcle-like behaviors of all of the following types of matter except:
   a. Subatomic particles
   b. X-Rays
   c. Soundwaves
   d. Electrons
   e. Photons

10. Which symbol illustrates a qubit?
    a. Ψ
    b. ∑
    c. B
    d. μ
    e. ¥

11. In the quantum world, everything is expressed as a:
    a. Specific numerical value
    b. Probabilities
    c. Absolutes
    d. Waves
    e. Particles

12. Roentgen originally described the x-ray photon as having ______-like movement.
    a. Mirror
    b. Particle
    c. Wave
    d. Visible light
    e. Atom

13. The Uncertainty Principle states what interferes with the measurement of a system?
    a. The measurement process
    b. Velocity of the particle being measured
    c. Position of the particle being measured
    d. State of the particle being measured
    e. Distance of one particle to another particle

14. If a photon does not have sufficient energy to penetrate a barrier, quantum mechanics allows the photon to tunnel underneath and reappear on the other side through:
    a. Quantum superposition
    b. Quantum computing
    c. Quantum observation
    d. Quantum tunneling
    e. Quantum entanglement

15. What is the result of Schrodinger's Cat experiment where the result is that the cat is simultaneously alive or dead depending on when the observation is made?
    a. Quantum superimposition
    b. Quantum computing
    c. Quantum tunneling
    d. Quantum entanglement

16. Quantum bits, or qubits, are shown similarly to bits in a 0 or 1 state. Qubits have the ability to be in a _________ state resulting in many more values.
    a. Steady
    b. Imposed
    c. Caffeinated
    d. Excited
    e. Superimposition

17. In 2023 the electron movement was described as 1 attosecond (as). One attosecond is equal to:
    a. 10^{-18} s
    b. 10^{2} s
    c. 10^{20} s
    d. 10^{-10} s
    e. 10^{16} s

18. What is the language of quantum physics?
    a. English
    b. Latin
    c. Greek
    d. Mandarin
    e. Mathematics

19. A qubit can be a:
    a. Photon
    b. Atom
    c. Electron
    d. All the answers
    e. None of the answers

20. Quantum computers will cause an increase in which functions in the future:
    a. Speed and accuracy
    b. Accuracy and capacity
    c. Speed and capacity
    d. Data storage and available space
    e. Available space and calculations

Worksheet 30-1
Digital Image Perception

Image perception has always been a distinct challenge for fluoroscopy. It returns in this 21st century as a challenge to the interpretation of digital medical images.

Image perception is a scientific term for what we call visual **sensitivity**. Image perception in medical imaging relates to how well we can visualize an image and although the radiologic technologist (RT) is not normally involved in image interpretation, it is the RT's responsibility to produce a quality image that can be properly interpreted.

Image perception is the visual sensitivity required for proper image interpretation. Fluoroscopic images are relatively dim, low intensity, and exhibit low contrast. Therefore the perception of anatomy is restricted by human visual anatomy.

1. The RT is responsible for producing a quality medical image with attention to each of the following except:
   a. Contrast resolution
   b. Image artifacts
   c. Image noise
   d. Spatial resolution
   e. Temporal resolution

2. The concept of *image perception* is closest in meaning to which of the following terms?
   a. Contrast resolution
   b. Spatial resolution
   c. Visual acuity
   d. Visual sensitivity
   e. Visual specificity

3. When the radiologist interprets an image to be abnormal and the image is later shown to be normal, how is that interpretation labeled?
   a. False negative
   b. False positive
   c. True negative
   d. True positive
   e. Visual accommodation

4. What results because of the entrance of the optic nerve on the retina?
   a. Blind spot
   b. Cones only vision
   c. Foveal vision
   d. Peripheral vision
   e. Visual search

5. How do we measure digital image illumination?
   a. Illumen
   b. Lumen
   c. Lux
   d. Search
   e. Sensitivity

6. An important part of the eye is the fovea centralis. What happens there?
   a. Low light vision
   b. Photopic vision
   c. Rod abundance
   d. Scotopic vision
   e. Visual cortex

7. Digital medical images should be visualized under what range of illumination?
   a. 10^0 – 10^1 lux
   b. 10^1–10^2 lux
   c. 10^2–10^3 lux
   d. 10^3–10^4 lux
   e. $>10^4$ lux

8. How can we best describe image interpretation by a radiologist?
   a. Foveal vision followed by peripheral vision
   b. Global impression followed by visual search
   c. Peripheral vision followed by foveal vision
   d. Production, processing, and prominent
   e. Visual search followed by a global impression

9. When the radiologist interprets an image to be normal and in fact the image is later shown to be abnormal, how is that interpretation labelled?
   a. False negative
   b. False positive
   c. Global impression
   d. True negative
   e. True positive

10. The ability to perceive small objects in an image is:
    a. Better with cones than rods
    b. Better with rods than cones
    c. Called contrast resolution
    d. Called contrast sensitivity
    e. Called wavelength sensitivity

11. The concept of *visual training* is the knowledge required for the:
    a. Medical physicist
    b. Radiologic technologist
    c. Radiologist
    d. Radiologist and radiologic technologist
    e. Radiologist, radiologic technologist, and medical physicist

12. What is an appropriate description of *foveal vision*?
    a. Best visual acuity
    b. Dim image
    c. High contrast image
    d. Image search
    e. Peripheral vision

13. One lumen per square meter is one
    a. Cone
    b. Illumen
    c. Illux
    d. Lux
    e. Rod

14. JND explains why it is easier to see a tissue mass on the mammogram of a fatty breast when compared to that of a dense breast. For what does JND stand?
    a. Jaundice never detected
    b. Joule not determined
    c. Joule noticed development
    d. Just not deep
    e. Just noticeable difference

15. Image illumination refers to what positive aspect of a digital medical image?
    a. Acuity
    b. Brightness
    c. Contrast
    d. Resolution
    e. Sensitivity

16. Protective eyewear is available for radiation protection. Which of the following also provides protection for the eye?
    a. Cornea
    b. Fovea
    c. Iris
    d. Pupil
    e. Retina

17. Rod instead of cone vision is associated with which of the following vision descriptors?
    a. Best visual acuity
    b. Blind spot
    c. High contrast and motion
    d. Low contrast and static
    e. Visual search

18. Dark adaptation by a radiologist before entering the dimly lit reading room is necessary to accommodate what visual aspect of human physiology?
    a. Cone-to-rod vision
    b. Iris size
    c. Pupil size
    d. Rod to cone vision
    e. Visual adaptation

19. Which of the following is the approximate maximum safe brightness for the human eye?
    a. 10^0 lux
    b. 10^1 lux
    c. 10^2 lux
    d. 10^3 lux
    e. 10^4 lux

20. Approximately how long does it take the human eye to focus on an image on a digital display device?
    a. 1 ms
    b. 10 ms
    c. 100 ms
    d. 200 ms
    e. 2000 ms

Worksheet 30-2 Receiver Operating Characteristics Curves

Receiver operating characteristic (ROC) attempts to evaluate various areas of decision-making. Image quality is most important because it determines how well digital image information is conveyed to the radiologist. This concept of conveyance as well as the skill of the radiologist can be evaluated with ROC curves.

Sensitivity and specificity are the basic measures of accuracy of a diagnostic test; however, they depend on the cut point used to define "positive" and "negative" test results. As the cut point shifts, sensitivity and specificity shift. The ROC curve is a plot of the sensitivity of a test versus its false-positive rate for all possible cut points. The advantages of the ROC curve as a means of defining the accuracy of a test, construction of the ROC, and identification of the optimal cut point on the ROC curve.

1. Artificial intelligence will likely improve interpretation time principally by shortening:
   a. Decision resolution
   b. Fixation time
   c. Global impression
   d. Temporal resolution
   e. Visual search

2. What is the single principal advantage of digital imaging over the previous analog imaging?
   a. Artifact reduction
   b. Contrast resolution
   c. Postprocessing
   d. Preprocessing
   e. Spatial resolution

3. *Sensitivity* is defined as:
   a. False negative fraction
   b. False positive fraction
   c. Total negative fraction
   d. True negative fraction
   e. True positive fraction

4. ROC curves are currently used in all the following areas except:
   a. Biometrics
   b. Machine learning
   c. Merchandizing
   d. Meteorology
   e. Weather forecasting

5. Total guessing would result in an area under the curve (AUC) of:
   a. 0%
   b. 25%
   c. 50%
   d. 75%
   e. 100%

6. Ergonomics requires the quality control technologist to have some metric data knowledge of each of the following except:
   a. Illumination
   b. Noise
   c. Temperature
   d. Work schedule
   e. Workstation

7. Accuracy as reported by the ROC curve is the value of:
   a. AUC
   b. (TP)/(TN)
   c. (TP)/(TN+FN)
   d. (TP+TN)/(FP+FN)
   e. (TP+TN)/(TP+TN+FP+FN)

8. Which of the following is associated with a misdiagnosis?
   a. Decision positive
   b. Decision threshold
   c. False positive
   d. Missed positive
   e. Positive position

9. *Sensitivity* is defined as the true positive rate (TPR). It could also properly be termed:
   a. Classified probability
   b. Conditional probability
   c. Cumulative probability
   d. Probability of abnormality
   e. Probability of detection

10. *Specificity* is defined as:
    a. False negative fraction
    b. False positive fraction
    c. Total negative fraction
    d. True negative fraction
    e. True positive fraction

11. Which of the following occupations do you think should have the most knowledge of ergonomics?
    a. Chef
    b. Medical physicist
    c. Office furniture salesperson
    d. Radiologic technologist
    e. Radiologist

12. If every interpretation of a medical image was wrong, the ROC AUC would be:
    a. 0%
    b. 25%
    c. 50%
    d. 75%
    e. 100%

13. An RT assigned to a workstation should exercise the 20-20-20 rule which is:
    a. Do 20 stretches at 20 meters within 20 minutes.
    b. Do 20 stretches within 20 minutes every 20 minutes.
    c. Every 20 minutes do 20 stretches while standing 20 minutes.
    d. Every 20 minutes look 20 feet away for 20 seconds.
    e. Every 20 minutes walk 20 feet away for 20 seconds

14. The sliding *decision threshold* has which of the following properties?
    a. Binary distribution
    b. Normal always less than abnormal
    c. Normal distribution
    d. Poisson distribution
    e. 10%–90% range

15. The false positive could also be properly termed:
    a. An abnormality
    b. A preexisting condition
    c. As detection
    d. A false alarm
    e. Normal tissue

16. An ROC curve is a
    a. Linear-linear plot of TPFversus FPF
    b. Linear-linear plot of TPF versus TNF
    c. Linear-log plot of TPF versus FPF
    d. Linear-log plot of TPF versus TNF
    e. Linear-log plot of TNF versus TPF

17. The concept of ROC curves was developed and used for many years in what industry prior to medical imaging?
    a. Individual sports
    b. Nuclear power
    c. Radio electronics
    d. Team sports
    e. Trucking

18. The value of (1-specificity) is the
    a. AUC
    b. False negative fraction (FNF)
    c. False positive fraction (FPF)
    d. True negative fraction (TNF)
    e. True positive fraction (TPF)

19. Ergonomics is best described by which of the following?
    a. Combining Integrating the Healthcare Enterprise and picture archiving and communication system
    b. Combining image to workstation
    c. Matching RT to image modality
    d. Matching radiologist to workstation
    e. Matching worker to work environment

20. The single most important metric on a ROC curve is
    a. AUC
    b. FNF
    c. FPF
    d. TNF
    e. TPF

Worksheet 31-1
Human Radiation Response
Composition of the Body

An understanding of how radiation affects biologic tissue is essential to the radiologic technologist's task of producing high-quality x-ray images with a minimum of radiation exposure. The composition of the human body has its basis in atoms, and it is at the atomic level that radiation interacts.

The atomic composition of the body determines the character and degree of the radiation interaction, and molecular and tissue composition defines the nature of the radiation response.

The following list summarizes the atomic composition of the body and shows that more than 85% of the body is hydrogen and oxygen.

- 0.1% phosphorus
- 0.1% sulfur
- 0.2% calcium
- 0.8% trace elements
- 2.4% nitrogen
- 10.7% carbon
- 25.7% oxygen
- 60.0% hydrogen

EXERCISES

1. The effects of fetal irradiation include all of the following *except:*
   a. Childhood malignancy
   b. Congenital malformation
   c. Diminished growth and development
   d. Erythema
   e. Neonatal death

2. Which of the following human responses to ionizing radiation would be categorized as a stochastic effect?
   a. Central nervous system syndrome
   b. Gastrointestinal syndrome
   c. Leukemia
   d. Extremity damage
   e. Hematologic depression

3. Most radiobiologic research is conducted with animals. Approximately how many human population groups have shown radiation effects?
   a. None
   b. Fewer than 5
   c. 5 to 10
   d. 10 to 20
   e. More than 20

4. Human responses to radiation that do *not* have a threshold dose are called:
   a. Large effects
   b. Stochastic effects
   c. Latent response
   d. Law effects
   e. Deterministic effects

5. Which of the following is the first step in producing a radiation response?
   a. Ionization
   b. Latent effect
   c. Manifestation of a lesion
   d. Molecular alteration
   e. Removal and isolation of a lesion

6. Approximately what percentage of the body is water?
   a. 20
   b. 35
   c. 50
   d. 65
   e. 80

7. Which element is *most* abundant in the body?
   a. Calcium
   b. Carbon
   c. Hydrogen
   d. Nitrogen
   e. Oxygen

8. Which molecule is *most* abundant in the body?
   a. Carbohydrate
   b. Lipid
   c. Nucleic acid
   d. Protein
   e. Water

9. A radiation effect that increases in severity with an increase in dose is called a:
   a. Stochastic effect
   b. Deterministic effect
   c. Late effect
   d. Delayed effect
   e. DNA

10. There are two main categories that we use to describe radiation damage. What are these categories called?
   a. Mitosis effect/meiosis effect
   b. Late effect/early effect
   c. Stochastic effect/deterministic effect
   d. Close effect/far-away effect
   e. Low-dose effect/high-dose effect

11. The stochastic effects of radiation on humans include effects that have these characteristics:
   a. Linear; threshold dose
   b. Nonlinear; threshold dose
   c. Linear; nonthreshold dose
   d. Nonlinear; nonthreshold dose
   e. None of the above

12. Radiation damage:
   a. Only can be observed immediately
   b. Can be observed only after years of waiting
   c. Cannot be repaired
   d. Can be observed only in humans
   e. Can be repaired at each stage in the damage sequence

13. An ionization event occurs:
   a. After telophase
   b. When an electron moves to an outer orbital shell
   c. When an atom loses an electron, potentially resulting in the breaking of a chemical bond
   d. While a ribosome is eating a lysosome
   e. At all phases of the cell cycle

14. *ALARA* stands for:
   a. As Long As Rooms Are Available
   b. As Low As Reasonably Achievable
   c. As Low As Responsibly Achievable
   d. As Long As Resting Allows
   e. None of the above

15. Which one of the following is not a deterministic effect of radiation?
   a. Lymphoma
   b. Skin erythema
   c. Lymphocyte depression
   d. Skin desquamation
   e. All of the above

16. A scientist who studies the effects of ionizing radiation on the body is called a/an:
   a. Medical physicist
   b. Radiologist
   c. X-ray technologist
   d. Radiation biologist
   e. Molecular biologist

Worksheet 31-2 Cell Theory

To understand the effects of radiation on the human body, one must have a basic knowledge of the composition and function of cells. The cell is considered the biologic building block. Every organ and tissue structure in the body is composed of many cells. Radiation injury begins when the cell is injured; therefore an understanding of cellular components and roles is important to understand how radiation damage occurs.

The single most important cellular component and molecule in the body is deoxyribonucleic acid (DNA). DNA contains all of the genes and is responsible for controlling the body's growth, development, and function.

It is assumed that the principal type of radiation damage is inflicted on the cell's control center—the DNA—and results in errors in metabolism that can produce a visible radiation effect.

EXERCISES

1. Anton van Leeuwenhoek:
   a. Accurately described a living cell in 1673 on the basis of microscopic observations
   b. Described atoms as having eyes and hooks
   c. Described the molecular structure of DNA in 1953
   d. First named the cell in 1665
   e. Showed conclusively that all plants and animals contain cells as their basic functional units

2. Schleiden and Schwann:
   a. Accurately described a living cell in 1673 on the basis of microscopic observations
   b. Described the molecular structure of DNA in 1953
   c. Developed the original periodic table
   d. First named the cell in 1665
   e. Showed conclusively that all plants and animals contain cells as their basic functional units

3. Watson and Crick:
   a. Accurately described a living cell in 1673 on the basis of microscopic observations
   b. Described the molecular structure of DNA in 1953
   c. Discovered x-ray crystallography
   d. First named the cell in 1665
   e. Showed conclusively that all plants and animals contain cells as their basic functional units

4. The production of large molecules from small ones is called:
   a. Anabolism
   b. Catabolism
   c. Hormesis
   d. Metabolism
   e. Mitosis

5. Which of the following are present in all tissues of the body and are the structural components of cell membranes?
   a. Carbohydrates
   b. Lipids
   c. Nucleic acids
   d. Proteins
   e. Sugars

6. The chief function of carbohydrates in the body is to:
   a. Assist in maintaining body temperature
   b. Exercise regulatory control over functions such as growth and metabolic rate
   c. Provide a defense mechanism against infection and disease
   d. Provide fuel for cell metabolism
   e. Provide structure and support

7. Which of the following is the concept of the relative constancy of the internal environment of the human body?
   a. Homeostasis
   b. Hormesis
   c. Meiosis
   d. Molecular composition
   e. Radiation hormesis

8. RNA:
   a. Contains all the hereditary information that represents a cell
   b. Is a principal component of a hormone
   c. Is located principally in the cytoplasm of the cell
   d. Is located principally in the nucleus of the cell
   e. Serves as the command or control molecule for all functions

9. Which of the following is an example of a macromolecule?
   a. A free radical
   b. A lipid
   c. An amino acid
   d. Salt
   e. Water

10. The breaking down of macromolecules into water and carbon dioxide is:
   a. Anabolism
   b. Catabolism
   c. Homeostasis
   d. Hormesis
   e. Metabolism

11. Which of the following molecules is a protein?
   a. A lipid
   b. A nucleic acid
   c. A salt
   d. An amino acid
   e. An enzyme

12. Lipids are:
   a. Energy storehouses
   b. Electrical conductors
   c. Inorganic compounds
   d. Micromolecules
   e. The sites of protein synthesis

13. Lipids store which of the following?
   a. Antibodies
   b. Enzymes
   c. Fat
   d. Salt
   e. Sugar

14. Organic molecules are defined as molecules that contain:
   a. Calcium
   b. Carbon
   c. Nitrogen
   d. Oxygen
   e. Sulfur

15. Which of the following is a principal component of protein?
   a. Amino acid
   b. Enzyme
   c. Lipid
   d. Peptide bond
   e. Sugar

16. The general formula $(C_6H_{10}O_5)_n$ represents which of the following?
   a. Amino acids
   b. Polysaccharides
   c. Genes
   d. Nucleic acids
   e. Proteins

17. Polysaccharides are which of the following?
   a. Carbohydrates
   b. Free radicals
   c. Lipids
   d. Nucleic acids
   e. Proteins

18. Which of the following base pairs is allowed for DNA?
   a. Adenine-cytosine
   b. Adenine-guanine
   c. Cytosine-thymine
   d. Guanine-cytosine
   e. Thymine-guanine

19. Homeostasis refers to what property of the body?
   a. Atomic composition
   b. Constancy of the internal environment
   c. Molecular composition
   d. Resistance to radiation
   e. Water content

20. Which of the following is the nitrogenous organic base found in RNA but *not* in DNA?
   a. Adenine
   b. Cytosine
   c. Guanine
   d. Thymine
   e. Uracil

21. The nucleic acids of the cell:
   a. Are found only in the nucleus
   b. Are macromolecules
   c. Consist of DNA and RNA
   d. Have a backbone of peptide bonds
   e. Store energy

Worksheet 31-3 Human Cells Tissues and Organs

To understand the effects of radiation on the human body, one must have a basic knowledge of human anatomy and physiology. The body is an extremely organized system, but it is composed mostly of water. Radiation interactions at the atomic level are transferred through the various levels of organization and can result in visible radiation effects.

Understanding human cell division and the role of DNA helps to understand how and why radiation effects occur. The phases of cell division include:

1. **Prophase:** nucleus swells and DNA becomes more prominent, beginning to take structural form
2. **Metaphase:** chromosomes line up in the central area of the cell
3. **Anaphase:** each chromosome splits at the centromere, creating sister chromatids
4. **Telophase:** chromosomes disappear into a mass of DNA, and the cytoplasm divides into two parts

Different tissues and organs have different radiosensitivities, depending on the types of cells they are composed of. Radiation injuries tend to be more severe if a cell is injured when it is immature. Injury severity also depends on the type of cell damage and which part of the cell life cycle it is in.

EXERCISES

1. "Crossing over":
   a. Is a process that occurs during meiosis, resulting in changes in the genetic constitution and inheritable traits
   b. Is characterized by the disappearance of structural chromosomes into a mass of DNA
   c. Is the final phase of mitosis
   d. Is the period of cell growth between divisions
   e. Is the phase of the cell cycle during which the nucleus swells and the DNA becomes more prominent and begins to take structural form

2. Ribosomes:
   a. Are called the workhorses of the cell
   b. Are helpful in the control of intracellular contaminants
   c. Are sites of protein synthesis that are essential to normal function
   d. Are small, pealike sacs that are capable of digesting cellular fragments and even the cell itself
   e. Digest macromolecules to produce energy for the cell

3. Lysosomes:
   a. Are called the workhorses of the cell
   b. Are sites of protein synthesis that are essential to normal cellular function
   c. Contain enzymes capable of digesting cell fragments
   d. Deliver energy to target molecules
   e. Digest macromolecules to produce energy for the cell

4. During which of the following subphases of meiosis does each chromosome split at the centromere, so that two chromatids are connected by a fiber to the poles of the nucleus?
   a. Anaphase
   b. Metaphase
   c. Prophase
   d. Telophase
   e. None of the above

5. In the human cell:
   a. Both the cytoplasm and the nucleus are surrounded by membranes.
   b. Lysosomes contain nucleic acid.
   c. Macromolecules are digested in the ribosomes.
   d. Macromolecules are synthesized in the mitochondria.
   e. The DNA passes through the endoplasmic reticulum.

6. Which of the following is part of interphase?
   a. DNA synthesis phase
   b. G_0 phase
   c. Prophase
   d. Protein synthesis phase
   e. Telophase

7. At metaphase, the chromosomes:
   a. Are visible in the microscope
   b. Line up at the poles of the cell
   c. Ooze through the cellular membrane
   d. Remain dominant
   e. Split apart and replicate

8. At what phase in mitosis are the chromosomes *most* visible?
   a. Anaphase
   b. Interphase
   c. Metaphase
   d. Prophase
   e. Telophase

9. Messenger RNA (mRNA) moves from:
   a. Cytoplasm to mitochondria
   b. Cytoplasm to nucleus
   c. Nucleus to lysosome
   d. Nucleus to mitochondria
   e. Nucleus to ribosome

10. During which of the following subphases of meiosis do the chromosomes appear and line up along the equator of the nucleus?
    a. Anaphase
    b. Metaphase
    c. Prophase
    d. Telophase
    e. None of the above

11. Which of the following make(s) up the bulk of the cell and contain(s) all of the molecular components in great quantity?
    a. Cellular inclusions
    b. Cytoplasm
    c. Endoplasmic reticulum
    d. Membranes
    e. Nucleus

12. Which of the following searches the cytoplasm for the amino acid for which it is coded, attaches to that amino acid, and then carries it to the ribosome?
    a. A codon
    b. DNA
    c. mRNA
    d. The endoplasmic reticulum
    e. tRNA

13. Meiosis:
    a. Results in two cells with 46 chromosomes each
    b. Is the process of division and reduction that occurs in genetic cells
    c. Is the process of division that occurs in somatic cells
    d. Results in the formation of two genetically identical daughter cells that look precisely like the parent cell
    e. None of the above

14. The body is organized in such a way that:
    a. Differentiated cells are immature.
    b. Epithelial cells usually are found inside organs.
    c. Mature cells are called stem cells.
    d. Organs combine to form tissues.
    e. Tissues and organs form an organ system.

15. Which of the following tissues is most radiosensitive?
    a. Bone marrow
    b. Brain
    c. Thyroid
    d. Muscle
    e. Skin

16. The nucleolus in particular contains which of the following?
    a. Amino acids
    b. DNA
    c. Lipids
    d. Proteins
    e. RNA

Worksheet 32-1
Law of Bergonié and Tribondeau
Physical Factors That Affect Radiosensitivity

Linear energy transfer (LET) expressed in keV/μm is the rate at which energy is transferred from ionizing radiation to tissue. In general, high-LET radiation is more damaging than low-LET radiation.

Different types of ionizing radiation have different LET, and the efficiency for producing a given response is related to LET. Such efficiency is measured by the relative biologic effectiveness (RBE), which is determined experimentally.

$$\text{RBE} = \frac{\text{Dose of standard radiation necessary to produce a given effect}}{\text{Dose of test radiation necessary to produce the same effect}}$$

EXERCISES

1. Which of the following is a part of the law of Bergonié and Tribondeau?
   a. A fetus is less radiosensitive than an adult.
   b. Stem cells are radiosensitive.
   c. The more mature a cell is, the more radiosensitive it is.
   d. When metabolism is high, radiosensitivity is low.
   e. When the proliferation rate is high, so is the radioresistance.

2. The law of Bergonié and Tribondeau states that:
   a. Mature cells are more sensitive than stem cells.
   b. Metabolic activity results in radioprotection.
   c. Radiosensitivity increases with increasing hypoxia.
   d. Radiosensitivity increases with the proliferation rate.
   e. The older a cell is, the more radiosensitive it is.

3. The response of tissue to radiation is principally a function of which of the following?
   a. Dose
   b. Fractionation
   c. LET
   d. Oxygen enhancement ratio (OER)
   e. RBE

4. The RBE:
   a. Describes tissue radiosensitivity
   b. Increases as x-ray energy increases
   c. Is a descriptor of the type of radiation
   d. Is equal to 3 keV/μm for alpha particles
   e. Is equal to 3 keV/μm for diagnostic x-rays

5. The law of Bergonié and Tribondeau relates to which of the following?
   a. Radiocurability and tumor size
   b. Radioresistance and cell lethality
   c. Radioresistance and oxygenation
   d. Radiosensitivity and cellular differentiation
   e. Radiosensitivity and oxygenation

6. The RBE:
   a. Has a value of 1 to 100
   b. Is a ratio of effects needed to produce a given dose
   c. Is a ratio of effects produced at a given dose
   d. Is higher for high-LET radiation than for low-LET radiation
   e. Refers to the type of effect

7. LET is measured in which of the following?
   a. Gray
   b. keV/rad
   c. keV/μm
   d. rad
   e. rad/μm

8. Which of the following has the highest LET?
   a. Alpha particles
   b. Cobalt-60 gamma rays
   c. Diagnostic x-rays
   d. Neutrons
   e. Protons

9. Diagnostic x-rays have an RBE of:
   a. 0.5
   b. 1
   c. 2
   d. 3
   e. 10

10. Dose fractionation is less effective than a single dose because:
   a. Dose fractionation has a low LET.
   b. Dose fractionation has a low OER.
   c. Fractionated doses are lower.
   d. Recovery occurs between doses.
   e. The RBE is less.

11. The LET, OER, and RBE are interrelated. Therefore which of the following statements is *true?*
   a. Diagnostic x-rays are considered low LET and RBE and high OER.
   b. Diagnostic x-rays have a higher LET than cobalt-60 gamma rays.
   c. Diagnostic x-rays have an LET of 3.0 keV/μm and an OER of 3.
   d. High-LET radiation has low RBE.
   e. High-RBE radiation has high OER.

12. LET is useful for expressing radiation:
   a. Dose
   b. Production
   c. Quality
   d. Quantity
   e. Response

13. What is related to radiation protection as LET is related to radiobiology?
   a. Dose
   b. Quantity factor
   c. Radiation weighting factor (WR)
   d. Response
   e. Tissue weighting factor (WT)

14. Which of the following has the lowest LET?
   a. Alpha particles
   b. Cobalt-60 gamma rays
   c. Diagnostic x-rays
   d. Fast neutrons
   e. Protons

15. Dose protraction relates principally to which of the following?
   a. Dose
   b. Dose accumulation
   c. Dose integration
   d. Dose rate
   e. Dose response

16. Which of the following is considered a physical dose-modifying factor?
   a. Age
   b. Cell progression
   c. Dose protraction
   d. Oxygen
   e. Recovery

17. Which of the following factors has no influence on response to radiation exposure?
   a. Age
   b. Dose protraction
   c. Occupation
   d. Oxygen tension
   e. Sex

18. Dose fractionation is less effective than an equal single dose because of which of the following?
   a. Cellular recovery
   b. Oxygenation and proliferation
   c. RBE and LET
   d. Reduced LET
   e. Reduced OER

19. Why do we develop radiation dose-response relationships?
   a. To establish benefit-risk coefficients
   b. To establish estimates of diagnostic accuracy
   c. To predict the harmful effects of radiation at low doses
   d. To predict the therapeutic value of an occupational exposure
   e. To predict the value of a radiologic examination

Worksheet 32-2
Biologic Factors That Affect Radiosensitivity Radiation Dose-Response Relationships

Tissue irradiated in the presence of oxygen (aerobic) responds to radiation more than does tissue irradiated under reduced levels of oxygen or in the absence of oxygen (hypoxic, anoxic, or anaerobic). The magnitude of this ratio in response is called the **oxygen enhancement ratio (OER)**.

$$\text{OER} = \frac{\text{Radiation dose necessary to produce an effect under anaerobic conditions}}{\text{Radiation dose necessary to produce same effect under aerobic condition}}$$

Most radiobiologic research is designed to establish the nature of radiation dose-response relationships. Such relationships generally can be classified as **linear** or **nonlinear** and **threshold** or **nonthreshold**. Knowledge of the precise nature of the radiation dose-response relationship allows one to predict human response after a given dose of radiation.

EXERCISES

1. Radiation-induced damage in tissue:
   a. Is caused by interaction at the tissue level
   b. Is greater in the presence of oxygen
   c. Is greater with protracted delivery
   d. Is irreversible
   e. Results in only latent effects

2. When one considers the biologic modifying factors to radiation response:
   a. Age is a factor.
   b. Nitrogen pressure is a factor.
   c. Pharmaceutical agents are capable only of protection.
   d. Pharmaceutical agents are capable only of sensitization.
   e. Sex is a factor.

3. Why is the linear, nonthreshold dose-response relationship used as a model for radiation protection guides?
   a. Because a linear response is directly proportional to the dose
   b. Because in a nonthreshold dose-response relationship, any dose is expected to produce a response
   c. Because of ALARA (As Low As Reasonably Achievable)
   d. Because such guides are concerned exclusively with the deterministic effects of radiation exposure
   e. Because such guides are concerned exclusively with the stochastic effects of radiation exposure

4. The time in life least sensitive to radiation exposure is which of the following?
   a. Adulthood
   b. Childhood
   c. In utero
   d. Old age
   e. There is no least sensitive time.

5. Which of the following effects exhibits a threshold type of radiation dose-response relationship?
   a. Cataracts
   b. Leukemia
   c. Shortening of life span
   d. Lung cancer
   e. Thyroid cancer

6. When a radiation dose-response relationship intercepts the response axis at a positive value:
   a. That response is acute.
   b. That response is not related to radiation.
   c. The radiation has a high LET.
   d. The relationship is linear.
   e. The relationship is nonlinear.

7. Which of the ensuing effects follows a nonlinear, threshold type of dose-response relationship?
   a. Breast cancer
   b. Skin effects
   c. Leukemia
   d. Shortening of life span
   e. Prostate cancer

8. Dose limits are based on which type of radiation dose-response relationship?
   a. Linear, nonthreshold
   b. Linear, quadratic
   c. Linear, threshold
   d. Nonlinear, nonthreshold
   e. Nonlinear, threshold

9. The stochastic effects of diagnostic x-rays probably follow which type of radiation dose-response relationship?
   a. Linear, nonthreshold
   b. Linear, quadratic
   c. Linear, threshold
   d. Nonlinear, nonthreshold
   e. Nonlinear, threshold

10. A wide error bar on a graphic data point indicates which of the following?
    a. A late effect
    b. Great confidence
    c. High LET
    d. Little confidence
    e. Low LET

11. The OER:
    a. Has a maximum value of about 10
    b. Is higher for protons than for photons
    c. Is highest for high-LET radiation
    d. Is highest for low-LET radiation
    e. Is independent of LET

12. Which of the following is considered a biologic dose-modifying factor?
    a. Dose per fraction
    b. Dose protraction
    c. Geometry
    d. LET
    e. The oxygen effect

13. Which of the following have the highest OER?
    a. Alpha particles
    b. Cobalt-60 gamma rays
    c. Diagnostic x-rays
    d. Neutrons
    e. Protons

14. Humans are most sensitive to radiation:
    a. At no special time
    b. During childhood
    c. During old age
    d. During preconception
    e. In utero

15. When an irradiated cell dies before the next mitosis, this is called:
    a. Clonal death
    b. Cytogenetic death
    c. Interphase death
    d. Metaphase death
    e. Mitotic death

16. A linear, nonthreshold dose-response relationship:
    a. Describes most deterministic effects
    b. Has a maximum response followed by a minimum response
    c. Is shaped like an "S"
    d. States that there is a range of very low doses that are totally safe
    e. Suggests that even the smallest dose may be risky

17. When a linear, nonthreshold dose-response relationship intersects the response axis at zero dose, this means that:
    a. It is not really linear.
    b. It is really threshold.
    c. Recovery and repair have occurred.
    d. There is a natural incidence of the response.
    e. There is no natural incidence of the response.

Worksheet 33-1 Molecular Radiobiology

When irradiated in vitro (outside the body), molecules are relatively resistant to radiation damage. However, when irradiated in vivo (inside the body), even relatively minor molecular damage can produce visible and sometimes significant effects at the whole-body level.

Irradiation of macromolecules can result in main-chain scission, cross-linking, or point lesions. The macromolecule of principal importance in vivo is DNA.

Irradiation of water produces free radicals, hydrogen peroxide (H_2O_2), and the hydroperoxyl radical (HO_2), each of which is considered a harmful molecular byproduct.

If radiation interacts with a macromolecule of importance, the subsequent effect is said to be **direct**. Alternatively, if radiation interacts with water, thereby creating one of the harmful byproducts, which then diffuses through the cell to the macromolecule, the effect is said to be **indirect**.

EXERCISES

1. After a low radiation dose, most cellular radiation damage that results in a late total-body effect occurs because of which of the following?
   a. Cross-linking
   b. In vitro effects
   c. Main-chain scission
   d. Point lesions
   e. Reduced viscosity

2. The biologically reactive molecular byproducts formed during radiolysis of water are thought to be which of the following?
   a. H_2O
   b. H* and OH*
   c. O_2 and H_2
   d. O and H
   e. SH compounds

3. Which of the following is the most radiosensitive molecule?
   a. DNA
   b. tRNA
   c. mRNA
   d. Ribosomes
   e. H_2O

4. Which of the following may occur in DNA molecules as a result of irradiation?
   a. Free radical formation
   b. Hydrogen bond breakage
   c. H_2O_2 formation
   d. A double-strand break
   e. Peroxy radical formation

5. When water is irradiated, the products of the *initial* interaction are which of the following?
   a. H_2O_2
   b. H_2O and e^-
   c. HOH^+ and e^-
   d. OH* and e^-
   e. OH* and H*

6. Which of the following is an example of anabolism?
   a. Hormesis
   b. Main-chain scission
   c. Protein synthesis
   d. Radiolysis of water
   e. Transfer RNA

7. Radiation-induced changes in DNA that result in genetic damage follow which type of dose-response relationship?
   a. Linear, nonthreshold
   b. Linear, quadratic
   c. Linear, threshold
   d. Nonlinear, nonthreshold
   e. Nonlinear, threshold

8. Which of the following is a free radical?
   a. e^-
   b. H_2O_2
   c. HO_2*
   d. HOH^+
   e. HOH^-

9. When molecules are irradiated:
   a. Directly, it is with x-rays
   b. In solution in vitro, they are in free radicals
   c. In suspension, they are irradiated in solution
   d. In suspension, they are irradiated in vivo
   e. Inside the cell or body, they are irradiated in vitro

10. Radiation effects at the total-body level occur mainly because of which of the following?
    a. Alterations in viscosity
    b. Direct effect
    c. Increased radiosensitivity
    d. Indirect effect
    e. Irradiation in vitro

Ionization of water yields the following:

$$H_2O + \text{Energy} \rightarrow H_2O^+ + e^-$$

H_2O^+ is unstable and instantly produces two subunits as follows:

$$\underset{(A)}{H_2O^+} \rightarrow \underset{(B)}{H^+} + \underset{(C)}{OH^*}$$

and

$$\underset{(D)}{H_2O^+} + \underset{(E)}{e^-} \rightarrow \underset{(F)}{H_2O^-}$$

followed by

$$\underset{(G)}{H_2O^-} \rightarrow \underset{(H)}{H^*} + \underset{(I)}{OH^-}$$

Match the ionization products given above (labeled A through I) with the description below in Questions 11 to 15

11. Which of the above is the hydrogen ion?
    a. A
    b. B
    c. C
    d. H
    e. I

12. Which of the above is the hydroxyl free radical?
    a. B
    b. C
    c. G
    d. H
    e. I

13. Which of the above is positively ionized water?
    a. A
    b. B
    c. C
    d. D
    e. F

14. Which of the above is the hydroxyl ion?
    a. B
    b. C
    c. G
    d. H
    e. I

15. Which of the above is the hydrogen-free radical?
    a. E
    b. F
    c. G
    d. H
    e. I

16. Of the various macromolecules that are sensitive to radiation, the most sensitive is/are:
    a. DNA
    b. Free radicals
    c. Proteins
    d. RNA
    e. Water

17. Which of the following is an effect of radiation on molecular DNA?
    a. Cross-linking
    b. Free radical formation
    c. H_2O_2 formation
    d. Increased viscosity
    e. The induction of radioactivity

Worksheet 34-1 Cellular Radiobiology

Radiation effects at the total-body level occur because of radiation damage to cells. Cellular damage, in turn, occurs because of molecular responses to radiation.

It is thought that certain critical molecules constitute sensitive targets within the cell, each of which must be inactivated to produce the ultimate response—cell lethality. This is the **target theory**.

The radiation dose-response relationship for cell lethality is **nonlinear** and **nonthreshold**. Cell survival follows the single-target, single-hit model or the multitarget, single-hit model of radiation-induced lethality. These models are the consequence of target theory and incorporate parameters useful for measuring the efficiency of various conditions of irradiation and the sensitivity of different types of cells.

D_{37} = Radiation dose after which 37% of cells will survive, whereas conversely, 63% will die
D_0 = Mean lethal dose; similar to D_{37} but applicable only to the straight-line portion of the multitarget, single-hit model
n = Extrapolation number
D_Q = Threshold dose or shoulder dose

EXERCISES

1. Which of the following phases of the cell cycle is considered *most* resistant?
   a. Early S phase
   b. G_1 phase
   c. G_2 phase
   d. Late S phase
   e. M phase

2. When cell-survival curves are used, the measure of cell radiosensitivity is which of the following?
   a. D_0
   b. D_Q
   c. n
   d. O_{37}
   e. RBE

3. When irradiated with high-LET radiation, human cells follow which of the following models?
   a. The linear, quadratic model
   b. The multitarget, multihit model
   c. The multitarget, single-hit model
   d. The single-target, multihit model
   e. The single-target, single-hit model

4. The probability of human cell death can be computed:
   a. If only D_0 is known
   b. If only D_Q is known
   c. If only n is known
   d. Using the normal distribution
   e. Using the Poisson distribution

5. If a dose equal to D_{37} were *uniformly* distributed, what percentage of cells would survive?
   a. 0%
   b. 37%
   c. 50%
   d. 63%
   e. 100%

6. Which of the following is the mean lethal dose?
   a. D_0
   b. D_Q
   c. D_{37}
   d. D_n
   e. n

7. The multitarget, single-hit model:
   a. Contains D_0, which is the threshold dose
   b. Contains n, which is the mean lethal dose
   c. Is characterized by D_{37}
   d. Is not a part of target theory
   e. Presumes a threshold

8. The difference in generation time among different types of cells is due mainly to the length of which of the following?
   a. The G_1 phase
   b. The G_2 phase
   c. The G_0 phase
   d. The M phase
   e. The S phase

9. Which of the following factors does *not* affect the radiation response of mammalian cells?
   a. Dose rate
   b. LET
   c. Presence of oxygen
   d. Sex of the cell
   e. Stage of the cell in its cycle

10. According to the multitarget model of cell lethality:
    a. Cells have more than one critical target, each of which has to be inactivated for cell death.
    b. Cells have one critical target and several secondary targets.
    c. Only cell death can be measured with accuracy.
    d. The cell can accumulate radiation dose.
    e. The critical target is considered to be the RNA.

11. In the following graph showing two survival curves, which of the following is *true?*

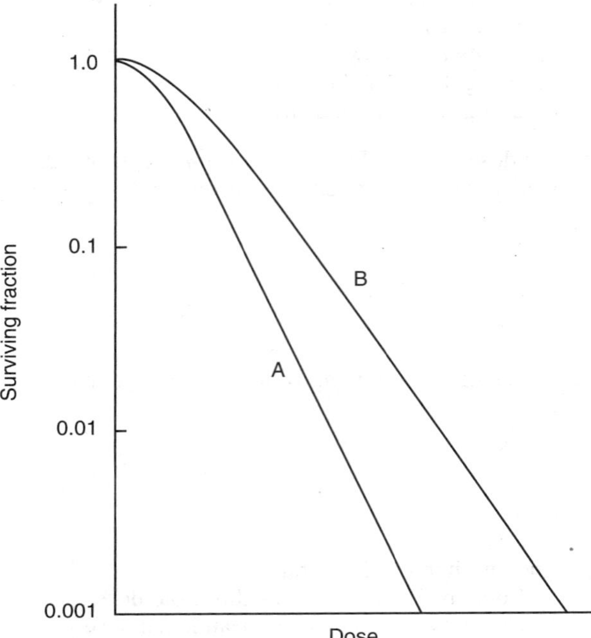

    a. Both curves have the same D_{37}.
    b. Both curves have the same D_Q.
    c. Both curves have the same mean lethal dose.
    d. Curve A could represent oxygenated cells if curve B represented anoxic cells.
    e. Curve A could represent protracted exposure if curve B represented single exposure.

12. According to target theory:
    a. A hit can occur only by direct effect.
    b. A hit can occur only by indirect effect.
    c. Radiation favors the target molecule.
    d. Radiation interacts randomly.
    e. Radiation interacts uniformly.

13. When irradiated with x-rays, human cells follow which of the following models?
    a. The linear, quadratic model
    b. The multitarget, multihit model
    c. The multitarget, single-hit model
    d. The single-target, multihit model
    e. The single-target, single-hit model

14. To explain radiation effects on living cells, target theory states that:
    a. A target can receive a hit by direct or indirect effect.
    b. Once hit, targets can be replaced.
    c. Only one target exists within the cell.
    d. Only one target must be hit to cause cell death.
    e. There is only one type of target.

15. If a dose equal to D_{37} were randomly distributed, what percentage of cells would die?
    a. 0%
    b. 37%
    c. 50%
    d. 63%
    e. 100%

16. Free radical ions are associated with biologic injury induced by which of the following types of radiation?
    a. Diagnostic x-rays
    b. Laser radiation
    c. Microwave radiation
    d. Radiofrequency
    e. Ultrasound

17. If undifferentiated cells are irradiated in vivo, such cells are:
    a. Difficult to replace
    b. Easy to replace
    c. Resistant to radiation
    d. Sensitive to radiation
    e. Very abundant

Worksheet 35-1 Acute Radiation Lethality Local Tissue Damage

The degree of radiation effect is related to the radiation dose and is predicted by a dose-response relationship. These conclusions are drawn from experimentation with animals and observations of humans irradiated both accidentally and intentionally.

Effects of radiation exposure at the whole-body level that occur within weeks of exposure are referred to as acute, or early, effects of radiation exposure. These effects include radiation lethality and radiation effects on local tissues. They are generally due to the death of many cells within the tissue.

EXERCISES

1. The $LD_{50/60}$ for humans is closest to which of the following?
   a. 1.6 Gy_t
   b. 2.5 Gy_t
   c. 3.5 Gy_t
   d. 4.5 Gy_t
   e. 6.0 Gy_t

2. A whole-body dose equivalent of 30 Gy_t would probably cause death in 4 to 10 days by which of the following mechanisms?
   a. Central nervous system death
   b. Gastrointestinal death
   c. Hemopoietic death
   d. Latent effects
   e. Prodromal syndrome

3. With regard to the radiation exposure of mammalian gonads:
   a. A linear, nonthreshold dose-response relationship prevails for sterility.
   b. Effects are apparently independent of linear energy transfer.
   c. Spermatocyte depression has been measured at as low as 0.1 Gy_t.
   d. Sterility is induced at doses as low as 0.5 Gy_t.
   e. The spermatocyte represents the most sensitive stage in the male.

4. The minimum testicular dose for transient infertility is approximately:
   a. 0.05 Gy_t
   b. 0.1 Gy_t
   c. 0.5 Gy_t
   d. 2.0 Gy_t
   e. 5.0 Gy_t

5. The $LD_{50/60}$ refers to a:
   a. Lethal dose delivered within 50 to 60 days
   b. Lethal dose of total-body radiation for 50% of the people so exposed in 60 days
   c. Lethal dose of total-body radiation for 50% to 60% of the people so exposed
   d. Lethal dose of total-body radiation for 50% of the people so exposed in 30 days
   e. Lethal dose for half the people younger than 50 years

6. The $LD_{50/60}$ represents the dose:
   a. Equivalent to 37% cell survival (D_{37})
   b. Required to kill 50% of the cells in 60 days
   c. Required to kill 60% of the cells in 50 days
   d. Resulting in 60% human death within 2 months
   e. That will kill half the people in 60 days

7. Human radiation lethality follows which dose-response relationship?
   a. Linear, quadratic
   b. Linear, nonthreshold
   c. Linear, threshold
   d. Nonlinear, nonthreshold
   e. Nonlinear, threshold

8. Which dose range, applied to both ovaries, is needed to induce permanent sterility?
   a. 0.1 to 1.0 Gy_t
   b. 1.0 to 2.0 Gy_t
   c. 2.0 to 5.0 Gy_t
   d. 5.0 to 12.0 Gy_t
   e. More than 12.0 Gy_t

9. Which syndrome has a mean survival time that is independent of dose?
   a. Central nervous system
   b. Gastrointestinal
   c. Hematologic
   d. Latent
   e. Prodromal

10. The dose of x-rays necessary to produce erythema in half of those exposed is approximately:
   a. 0.5 Gy_t
   b. 1.0 Gy_t
   c. 3.0 Gy_t
   d. 5.0 Gy_t
   e. 10.0 Gy_t

11. The acute radiation syndrome consists of all of the following *except:*
    a. Central nervous syndrome
    b. Gastrointestinal syndrome
    c. Hematologic syndrome
    d. Latent injury syndrome
    e. Latent period

12. Which of the following is *not* a deterministic response to radiation exposure?
    a. Breast cancer
    b. Chromosomal aberrations
    c. Epilation
    d. Intestinal distress that occurs 1 week after exposure
    e. Skin erythema that occurs 2 weeks after exposure

13. Which of the following is a delayed local tissue effect?
    a. Cataracts
    b. Epilation
    c. Moist desquamation
    d. Skin erythema
    e. Transient sterility

14. Five days after a whole-body dose of 10 Gy_t is received, physiologic alterations in the small intestine include all of the following *except:*
    a. Crypt cell death
    b. Diarrhea
    c. Epilation
    d. Leakage of proteins from the intestinal lumen
    e. Loss of electrolytes and water

15. Acute radiation syndrome:
    a. Begins at a threshold dose of 0.5 Gy_t
    b. Resulting in gastrointestinal death indicates a mean survival time of about 4 to 10 days
    c. Can occur after high doses administered over a short time or over several months
    d. Includes the gastrointestinal syndrome, which occurs after doses of approximately 50 to 100 Gy_t
    e. Includes the most sensitive of the syndromes—the gastrointestinal syndrome

16. The mean survival time after a lethal radiation dose is constant:
    a. Between 2.0 and 10.0 Gy_t
    b. For gastrointestinal death
    c. For hematologic death
    d. With increasing the dose to more than 50 Gy_t
    e. With increasing the dose to more than 100 Gy_t

17. Which of the following is considered a deterministic response to radiation exposure?
    a. Skin erythema
    b. Breast cancer
    c. Genetic damage
    d. Leukemia
    e. Shortened life span

18. The mean survival time for mammals after a single whole-body dose of radiation is:
    a. Dependent on dose ($\approx$2–10 Gy_t)
    b. Dependent on repair mechanisms
    c. Independent of dose
    d. Independent of the type of death
    e. The same for all species

19. Death caused by a single dose of total-body irradiation primarily involves damage to which of the following?
    a. Bone marrow
    b. Endocrine system
    c. Respiratory system
    d. Skeletal system
    e. Skin

Worksheet 35-2 Hematologic Effects Cytogenetic Effects

All of the acute radiation effects observed at the whole-body level have been studied thoroughly in experimental animals. Most have been observed in human populations, including atomic bomb survivors, radiation accident victims, and patients with radiation-induced cancer.

Blood is a body tissue that has received considerable attention as a biologic in vivo radiation dosimeter. Because blood is radiosensitive and is easy to sample, it is often used to predict the likely outcome of an unknown radiation exposure.

Cell counts and cytogenetic analysis of lymphocytes are conducted on all radiation accident victims to determine the aggressiveness of supportive therapy and to help guide treatment.

EXERCISES

1. Which of the following cell types is most severely depressed by radiation?
   a. Erythrocytes
   b. Granulocytes
   c. Lymphocytes
   d. Megakaryocytes
   e. Neurons

2. The normal human karyotype consists of:
   a. 23 chromosomes
   b. 23 chromosome pairs
   c. 42 autosomes
   d. 46 autosomes
   e. Two sex chromosome pairs

3. Of the following chromosomal aberrations, which requires a karyotype for analysis?
   a. Chromatid deletion
   b. Dicentric chromosome
   c. Isochromatid fragments
   d. Reciprocal translocation
   e. Ring chromosome

4. Which of the following blood observations is *most* appropriate during monitoring for radiation response?
   a. Erythrocyte count
   b. Granulocyte count
   c. Hematocrit
   d. Lymphocyte count
   e. Thrombocyte count

5. A whole-body radiation dose of 0.25 Gy_t is *most* likely to produce which of the following?
   a. Hematologic damage
   b. Depletion of oogonia
   c. Epilation
   d. Erythrocyte depression
   e. Skin erythema

6. Which of the following is *not* a mature blood cell?
   a. Cystocyte
   b. Erythrocyte
   c. Granulocyte
   d. Lymphocyte
   e. Thrombocyte

7. Radiation effects on the hematologic system:
   a. Are first observed as a lymphocyte depression
   b. Are measurable at whole-body doses as low as 5 rad
   c. Are permanent
   d. Cannot result in a late response
   e. Suggest that radiation workers should undergo routine blood analysis

8. Which of the following blood observations is *most* appropriate for routine monitoring of radiation workers?
   a. Erythrocyte count
   b. Lymphocyte count
   c. Shilling differential
   d. Thrombocyte count
   e. None of the above

9. Which of the following chromosomal aberrations obeys a linear, nonthreshold dose-response relationship?
   a. Chromatid break
   b. Dicentric chromosome
   c. Reciprocal translocation
   d. Ring chromosome
   e. Tricentric chromosome

10. Which cells are involved in the human immune response?
    a. Erythrocytes
    b. Granulocytes
    c. Lymphocytes
    d. Spermatocytes
    e. Thrombocytes

11. Which cells are *most* sensitive to radiation exposure?
   a. Cystocytes
   b. Erythrocytes
   c. Granulocytes
   d. Lymphocytes
   e. Thrombocytes

12. What phase of the cell cycle has the *most* variable length?
   a. G_0
   b. G_1
   c. G_2
   d. M
   e. S

13. Which of the following is the precursor to a thrombocyte?
   a. Cystocyte
   b. Lymphocyte
   c. Megakaryoblast
   d. Myeloblast
   e. Reticulocyte

14. Which two cell lines are the *most* radiosensitive?
   a. Granulocytes, lymphocytes
   b. Granulocytes, oogonia
   c. Granulocytes, spermatogonia
   d. Spermatogonia, lymphocytes
   e. Spermatogonia, oogonia

15. Which of the following human cells are *most* often used for cytogenetic analysis?
   a. Lymphocytes
   b. Oogonia
   c. Skin cells
   d. Spermatogonia
   e. Thrombocytes

16. How long after radiation exposure do chromosomal aberrations first appear in peripheral blood cells?
   a. Hours
   b. Months
   c. Years
   d. Decades
   e. Never

17. The principal response of the blood to radiation exposure is:
   a. A decrease in cell number
   b. Stimulation of cell proliferation
   c. Cellular transformation
   d. Fragmentation of chromosomes
   e. Rearrangement of chromosomes

18. After radiation exposure, the first blood cells to respond are the:
   a. Cystocytes
   b. Erythrocytes
   c. Granulocytes
   d. Lymphocytes
   e. Thrombocytes

19. A chromosomal karyotype is:
   a. A description of the radiation response
   b. A point mutation
   c. An analysis of chromosomal fragments
   d. An orderly map of chromosomes
   e. Unrestrained growth of chromosomes

20. Evidence suggests that the most harmful male genetic mutations occur in which of the following?
   a. Leydig cells
   b. Sertoli cells
   c. Spermatocytes
   d. Spermatids
   e. Postspermatogonia cells

Worksheet 36-1
Local Tissue Effects
Life Span Shortening
Risk Estimates

Delayed or late responses to radiation exposure are called stochastic effects and include genetic effects and somatic effects that require months or even years to develop. Radiobiologists rely heavily on data extrapolated from observations of humans who have suffered high radiation doses or on large-scale epidemiologic studies.

These stochastic effects generally follow low doses of radiation. Precise dose-response relationships are seldom possible to determine; therefore radiation scientists resort to various estimates of risk.

Principal stochastic effects of concern are the induction of malignant disease and genetic effects. Each of these is presumed to follow a linear, nonthreshold dose-response relationship. Late local tissue effects are for the most part threshold in nature.

EXERCISES

1. Which of the following is an example of a linear, nonthreshold, dose-response relationship?
   a. Cataracts
   b. CNS syndrome
   c. Epilation
   d. Lethality
   e. Leukemia

2. Which of the following statements about radiation-induced cataracts after a CT examination of the head is *most* appropriate?
   a. Cataracts are possible because there is no threshold.
   b. Lens shields should be used.
   c. The dose is probably below the threshold for such an effect.
   d. The dose is probably in the neighborhood of the threshold for such an effect.
   e. The probability of cataracts is high.

3. The best estimate for radiation-induced life span shortening is:
   a. 10 hours/10 mGy_t
   b. 10 days/10 mGy_t
   c. 24 hours/10 mGy_t
   d. 24 days/10 mGy_t
   e. 1 month/10 mGy_t

4. Diagnostic x-rays have been shown to produce which of the following?
   a. Cataracts
   b. Chromosomal aberrations
   c. Leukemia
   d. Organ atrophy
   e. Shortening of life

5. Supporting evidence for radiation carcinogenesis comes from:
   a. British radiologists
   b. Fluoroscopic monitoring of patients with tuberculosis
   c. ^{131}I therapy for hyperthyroidism
   d. Pelvimetry
   e. People living in areas with high background radiation (e.g., Denver)

6. If the incidence of cancer is 1:5000, what is the relative risk if an irradiated population shows an incidence of 4:10,000?
   a. 2:1
   b. 4:1
   c. 10:1
   d. 1000:1
   e. 4000:1

7. Which of the following groups has suffered a harmful radiation effect?
   a. Patients receiving diagnostic x-rays
   b. Nuclear power plant workers
   c. Radiologic technologists
   d. Radium watch-dial painters
   e. The last generation of radiologists

8. Radiation-induced cataracts:
   a. Appear on the posterior pole of the lens
   b. Exhibit a threshold to x-rays of approximately 10 rad
   c. Follow a linear, nonthreshold type of dose-response relationship
   d. Follow a nonlinear, threshold type of dose-response relationship
   e. Have a latent period of approximately 1 year

9. Approximately how many Americans will die of malignant disease from natural causes?
   a. 5%
   b. 10%
   c. 20%
   d. 40%
   e. 50%

10. Significant gonadal radiation exposure occurs:
    a. In whole-body MRI
    b. Only when no collimator is used
    c. When radiation is scattered from other parts of the body
    d. When radiation is scattered internally
    e. When the gonads are in the primary beam

11. Epidemiology is the study of which of the following?
    a. Early radiation effects
    b. Late radiation effects
    c. Populations
    d. Radiation
    e. Statistics

12. Radiation-induced chromosomal aberrations are which of the following?
    a. Early or late effects
    b. Observable following 5 mGy_t dose rad
    c. Only early effects
    d. Only late effects
    e. Present only after whole-body irradiation

13. The average latent period for radiation-induced cataracts is:
    a. 5 years
    b. 15 years
    c. 30 years
    d. 50 years
    e. Life

14. The approximate acute x-ray dose required to produce a 100% incidence of cataracts is:
    a. 1 Gy_t
    b. 10 Gy_t
    c. 100 Gy_t
    d. 1000 Gy_t
    e. 10,000 Gy_t

15. Which of the following has the greatest loss-of-life expectancy?
    a. Accidents
    b. Being male
    c. Cancer
    d. Occupation
    e. Radiation

16. Protective lens shields for patients should be used:
    a. Always
    b. Never
    c. When the lens is in the primary beam and such use does not interfere with the examination
    d. Whenever the lens is in the primary beam
    e. Not enough information is given.

17. Breast cancer is observed in 30 of 450 patients. If the normal incidence is 2:1000, what is the approximate relative risk in these patients?
    a. 10:1
    b. 30:1
    c. 50:1
    d. 100:1
    e. 300:1

Worksheet 36-2
Radiation-Induced Malignancy
Total Risk of Malignancy
Radiation and Pregnancy

It is undeniable that humans are most sensitive to the harmful effects of radiation while in utero. Furthermore, the fetus is most radiation sensitive early in pregnancy. Radiation effects include prenatal and postnatal mortality, congenital abnormalities, and latent malignant disease.

Low-dose irradiation (e.g., 0.1 Gy_t) has never caused such effects in humans. Only epidemiologic studies such as the Oxford survey have suggested an increased risk of latent malignant disease after low-dose in utero irradiation.

No direct evidence of radiation-induced genetic effects has been found in humans.

Observations of flies and mice, however, have shown the following:

1. Radiation-induced genetic mutations follow a linear, nonthreshold dose-response relationship.
2. The passage of time leads to some recovery from the genetic effects of radiation.
3. Radiation does not induce specific genetic mutations but rather increases the incidence of already existing mutations.
4. Radiation-induced genetic mutations are usually recessive.
5. For humans, the doubling dose is approximately 0.5 Gy_t.

EXERCISES

1. The relative risk of leukemia after low-dose irradiation in utero is approximately:
   a. 0.5
   b. 1.5
   c. 3.5
   d. 5.0
   e. 10

2. Radiation-induced leukemia:
   a. Can be reversed
   b. Does not occur after long-term, low-level radiation exposure
   c. Follows a linear, threshold dose-response relationship
   d. Has been demonstrated in both animals and humans
   e. Probably does not occur at doses of less than approximately 250 mSv

3. Which of the following dose-response relationships best describes radiation-induced lung cancer?
   a. Linear, nonthreshold
   b. Linear, quadratic
   c. Linear, threshold
   d. Nonlinear, nonthreshold
   e. Nonlinear, threshold

4. Which of the following numbers approximates the total cases of leukemia observed in the 100,000 atomic bomb survivors?
   a. 50
   b. 150
   c. 500
   d. 1500
   e. 5000

5. Which of the following statements about the development of radiation-induced liver cancer in Thorotrast-injected patients is *true?*
   a. The findings are negative.
   b. The findings are positive and statistically significant.
   c. The findings are positive but not statistically significant.
   d. The radiation source was iodine.
   e. The suspected principal radiation dose comes from beta emission.

6. After a dose of 100 mGy_t at 6 weeks of gestation, the increase in congenital abnormalities is approximately:
   a. 0.1%
   b. 1%
   c. 10%
   d. 25%
   e. 50%

7. The latent period of radiation-induced leukemia is considered to be:
   a. 1 year
   b. 1 to 3 years
   c. 4 to 7 years
   d. 8 to 12 years
   e. >12 years

8. Analysis of the survivors of the atomic bomb shows that the induction of leukemia:
   a. Does not exist
   b. Peaked 10 years after the bomb
   c. Principally implicates chronic lymphocytic leukemia
   d. Suggests a threshold of 3 Gy_td
   e. Supports a linear, nonthreshold dose-response relationship

9. Which of the following populations has shown an increased incidence of leukemia after radiation exposure?
   a. American radiologic technologists
   b. Atomic bomb survivors
   c. Chernobyl survivors
   d. Diagnostic imaging patients
   e. Radium watch-dial painters

10. Which of the following types of cancer has *not* been demonstrated in humans after irradiation?
    a. Breast
    b. Colon
    c. Liver
    d. Lung
    e. Skin

11. Which type of radiation-induced cancer exhibits a threshold dose-response relationship?
    a. Bone
    b. Breast
    c. Liver
    d. Lung
    e. Skin

12. The relative risk of leukemia after irradiation in utero:
    a. Is approximately 50
    b. Is approximately 100
    c. Is less than 1.0 at zero dose
    d. Would equal 1.0 if there were no risk
    e. Would equal 100 if there were no risk

13. Which of the following radiation responses in utero is *most* likely when exposure occurs during organogenesis?
    a. Childhood cancer
    b. Congenital abnormalities
    c. Leukemia
    d. Neonatal death
    e. Prenatal death

14. With regard to radiation-induced genetic mutations:
    a. The dose-response relationship is nonlinear.
    b. The dose-response relationship is threshold.
    c. The doubling dose is approximately 0.5 to 2.5 mGy_t.
    d. The male is more sensitive than the female.
    e. The most frequent types are dominant.

15. The data and conclusions of the Oxford survey:
    a. Are based on exposure of mice
    b. Show a 100% incidence of effects after an exposure of 2 Gy_t
    c. Suggest a relative risk of approximately 8:1 during the first trimester of pregnancy
    d. Suggest a threshold for cataracts of approximately 2 Gy_t
    e. Suggest a shortening of the life span by 10 days/10 mGy_t

Worksheet 37-1
Cardinal Principles of Radiation Protection
Dose Limits

Time and experience have led to a body of rules, regulations, and recommendations known as the principles of radiation protection. Exposure levels considered to be safe have been established, and these have been supplemented by the concept of **ALARA** (*as low as reasonably achievable*). Procedures and techniques have been developed to maintain occupational exposure below recommended limits and to ensure that all exposures are ALARA.

The cumulative **dose limit (DL)** is the dose that, if received each year during a 40-year occupational span, would result in an acceptable risk of injury.

Three principles of radiation control are known as the cardinal principles:

1. Keep the time of radiation exposure as short as possible.
2. Increase the distance from the source of radiation.
3. Place shielding between the radiation source and the person who is being shielded.

These cardinal principles of radiation protection must be applied. Nearly all of the protective procedures and devices that are used in diagnostic radiology incorporate some aspect of these principles.

EXERCISES

1. Half-value layer (HVL) is related to which of the following principles of radiation protection?
   a. Distance
   b. Exposure
   c. Monitoring
   d. Shielding
   e. Time

2. If all other factors remain constant, radiation dose is related to x-ray beam-on time:
   a. By the inverse square
   b. Directly
   c. Exponentially
   d. Geometrically
   e. Inversely

3. If all other factors remain constant, the radiation dose is related to source-to-object distance:
   a. By the inverse square
   b. Directly
   c. Exponentially
   d. Inversely
   e. Proportionately

4. If all other factors remain constant, radiation dose is related to shielding:
   a. By the inverse square
   b. Directly
   c. Exponentially
   d. Inversely
   e. Proportionately

5. One tenth-value layer (TVL) is defined as:
   a. $\frac{1}{10}$ the initial dose
   b. $\frac{1}{10}$ the initial shielding
   c. 10 times the HVL
   d. The shielding necessary to reduce exposure to $\frac{1}{10}$
   e. The shielding that will produce 10 times the dose

6. One TVL is equal to approximately how many HVLs?
   a. 2.0
   b. 2.2
   c. 3.3
   d. 5.0
   e. 10.0

7. During radiography, the best position for the radiologic technologist is:
   a. Behind the operating console barrier
   b. Down the hall
   c. Holding the patient
   d. In the examination room and as far from the patient as practical
   e. In the examination room and next to the patient

8. The HVL for 70 kVp is greater:
   a. For long exposure time than for short exposure time
   b. Than that for 90 kVp
   c. Than the TVL for 70 kVp
   d. With high filtration than with low filtration
   e. With single-phase power than with three-phase power

9. The exposure rate from a point source is 1 mGy_a/h at 120 cm. If a radiologic technologist moves to within 30 cm of the source of radiation, how many HVLs would be needed to reduce the exposure rate to 1 mGy_a/h?
   a. 1
   b. 2
   c. 4
   d. 6
   e. 8

10. If a survey meter reads 0.25 mGy/h, how long can a person stay at that location before receiving an exposure of 1 mGy?
    a. 1 hour
    b. 2 hours
    c. 4 hours
    d. 6 hours
    e. 8 hours

11. If the exposure rate 1 m from a source is 90 mGy/h, what is the exposure rate at 3 m from the source?
    a. 1 mGy/h
    b. 9 mGy/h
    c. 10 mGy/h
    d. 30 mGy/h
    e. 90 mGy/h

12. The exposure rate alongside a fluoroscopic table (distance = 60 cm from the source) is 4 mGy/h. Therefore if the radiologic technologist:
    a. Completed a 3-minute barium enema, the exposure would be 0.2 mGy.
    b. Completed a procedure at a distance of 120 cm, the total exposure would be 0.4 mGy.
    c. Completed a procedure that required 10 minutes, the exposure would be 0.4 mGy.
    d. Moved 60 cm farther from the table, the exposure rate would be 2 mGy/h.
    e. Moved 60 cm farther from the table, the exposure rate would be increased.

13. The occupational effective dose is assumed to be:
    a. <20% of monitored dose
    b. <10% of monitored dose
    c. <5% of monitored dose
    d. <10% of output dose
    e. <5% of output dose

14. A radiation exposure device (RED) is?
    a. A bomb that disperses radioactive material
    b. A bomb that produces a nuclear explosion
    c. A sealed source of radioactive material that directly exposes people
    d. An x-ray tube set at 120 kVp
    e. The color of most barns

15. During fluoroscopy, the exposure rate at the technologist's position is 3.5 mGy/hr. How much x-ray beam-on time is allowed before the technologist reaches 1 mGy?
    a. 8 minutes
    b. 17 minutes
    c. 35 minutes
    d. 1 hour
    e. 2 hours

16. Most occupational dose to radiographers occurs during which type of exam?
    a. Fluoroscopy
    b. X-ray
    c. Computed tomography
    d. Magnetic resonance imaging
    e. Ultrasound

17. Effective dose gives us an idea of what the equivalent ___________ dose would be.
    a. Liver
    b. Gonads
    c. Breast
    d. Lungs
    e. Whole body

Worksheet 38-1
Design of X-Ray Apparatus
Design of Protective Barriers

Designers of x-ray facilities and equipment exercise considerable care and attention. Much of this attention results from the need for radiation protection.

X-ray imaging systems have filters, collimators, and shields to reduce radiation exposure to patients and personnel. Attention is given to the proper design and calibration of kVp, mA, and exposure timers so that radiographic techniques can be accurately and consistently used. This accuracy reduces the number of reexaminations, which in turn reduces human exposure. This is why periodic radiation control surveys and performance evaluation of x-ray apparatus are recommended.

Nearly all diagnostic x-ray rooms have lead in the walls. Sometimes, floor and ceiling barriers also require lead shielding.

EXERCISES

1. Every diagnostic x-ray tube housing must be sufficiently shielded to limit the level of exposure 1 m from the housing to:
   a. 0.1 mGy_a/h
   b. 1 mGy_a/h
   c. 10 mGy_a/h
   d. A factor that varies according to kVp
   e. A factor that varies according to use

2. During mammography, at tube potentials less than 30 kVp, the minimum acceptable total equivalent filtration is:
   a. 0.05 mm Al
   b. 0.1 mm Al
   c. 0.25 mm Al
   d. 0.5 mm Al
   e. 2.5 mm Al

3. The minimum permissible filtration for general-purpose radiographic or fluoroscopic tubes is:
   a. 0.05 mm Al
   b. 0.1 mm Al
   c. 0.25 mm Al
   d. 0.5 mm Al
   e. 2.5 mm Al

4. The fluoroscopic tube should *not* be positioned closer than 38 cm to the tabletop because the:
   a. Bucky slot would interfere
   b. Geometric unsharpness would increase
   c. Heat load on the tube would increase
   d. Patient radiation dose would be excessive
   e. Resultant magnification would be objectionable

5. Which of the following is regulated in a controlled area?
   a. Patient flow
   b. Public access
   c. Radiation exposure
   d. Type of procedure
   e. X-ray operation

6. Radiographic workload (W) has units of:
   a. mAmin/wk
   b. mGy/mAmin
   c. mGy/mAs
   d. Gy/mAmin/wk
   e. Gy/wk

7. The radiographic workload in a busy radiography and fluoroscopy (RF) room is approximately:
   a. 10 mAmin/wk
   b. 50 mAmin/wk
   c. 100 mAmin/wk
   d. 500 mAmin/wk
   e. 5000 mAmin/wk

8. Which of the following locations in a hospital should have the highest occupancy factor (T)?
   a. Laboratory
   b. Elevator
   c. Corridor
   d. Restroom
   e. Waiting room

9. Which of the following usually is considered to be a secondary protective barrier?
   a. All walls
   b. Chest wall
   c. Control booth barrier
   d. Floor
   e. Lateral wall

10. Fluoroscopic x-ray units must:
    a. Be image-intensified
    b. Have at least 2.5 mm Al equivalent filtration
    c. Have spot-film capability
    d. Limit leakage radiation to 10 mGy_a/h at 1 m from the tube
    e. Never exceed 100 mGy_a/min at the tabletop

11. Which of the following contributes to the exposure of radiologic personnel?
    a. Off-focus radiation
    b. Primary radiation
    c. Remnant x-rays
    d. Scatter radiation
    e. Useful beam

12. The design limit for exposure of occupants in controlled areas is:
    a. 10 μSv/wk
    b. 0.1 mSv/wk
    c. 1 mSv/wk
    d. 5 mSv/wk
    e. 10 mSv/wk

13. The use factor (U):
    a. Applies only to radiography, not fluoroscopy
    b. Describes the use of the room
    c. Describes the use of the x-ray tube
    d. Is always 1 for secondary barriers
    e. Takes on values from 0 to 10

14. All fluoroscopes have a 5-minute reset timer:
    a. Because no patient shall ever receive more than 5 minutes of x-ray beam-on time
    b. To allow image receptor change
    c. To permit a tube cool-down period
    d. To protect the patient
    e. To protect the x-ray tube

15. A test to ensure that radiation intensity is doubled when radiographic mA is doubled is called a test of:
    a. Alignment
    b. Coincidence
    c. Linearity
    d. Reproducibility
    e. Uniformity

16. When the fluoroscopic x-ray tube is mounted farther under the table, what is reduced?
    a. Beam alignment
    b. Filtration
    c. Image receptor speed
    d. Patient dose
    e. Scatter radiation

17. Which of the following would definitely be a secondary barrier?
    a. All walls of a dedicated chestroom
    b. Any wall in a CT room
    c. The chest wall in an RF room
    d. The door
    e. The floor

18. What is the weekly workload if 20 patients are examined each day at an average of 78 kVp/60 mAs per view and 3.4 views per patient?
    a. 68 mAmin/wk
    b. 340 mAmin/wk
    c. 442 mAmin/wk
    d. 500 mAmin/wk
    e. >700 mAmin/wk

19. A dedicated chest examination room is used to image 40 patients per day, two views per patient, and the PA technique is 110 kVp/1.5 mAs; the LAT technique is 120 kVp/3 mAs. What is the workload?
    a. 5 mAmin/wk
    b. 15 mAmin/wk
    c. 30 mAmin/wk
    d. 65 mAmin/wk
    e. 100 mAmin/wk

Worksheet 38-2 Radiation Detection and Measurement

For many years, film was the only type of detector available to indicate the presence of x-radiation. As a radiation detector, photographic emulsion has many advantages, but it also has many disadvantages. Its advantages continue to qualify it for personnel radiation monitoring—the film badge.

Other methods of radiation detection and measurement are now available, and some of them are more sensitive, more accurate, and more applicable to certain situations.

Gas-filled detectors are used for x-ray output calibration and radiation monitoring of areas for exposure levels. Thermoluminescent dosimetry (TLD) and optically stimulated luminescence are used for personnel monitoring and patient dose estimation. Scintillation detectors are used principally in nuclear medicine imaging apparatuses such as the gamma camera.

Instruments that incorporate nearly all of these methods can be designed for many different uses. To apply the best possible instrumentation to a given situation, one must understand the basic operating principles of each method and the associated characteristics of sensitivity, accuracy, range, and type of radiation detected.

EXERCISES

1. Which of the following is a characteristic of the ionization chamber survey meter?
   a. Geiger-Müller counter
   b. Detection of individual ionizations
   c. Highly sensitive, 0.1 $\mu Gy_a/h$
   d. Narrow range, 10 μGy_a to 50 mGy_a/h
   e. Wide range, 10 μGy_a to 1000 mGy_a/h

2. Gas-filled radiation detectors are used:
   a. As a proportional counter to measure the output of an x-ray machine
   b. As an integration type of ionization chamber
   c. Because they are more sensitive than scintillation detectors
   d. For occupational radiation monitoring
   e. In the Geiger region to map the radiation exposure levels in fluoroscopy

3. If each stage of a photomultiplier tube has a gain of approximately 4, a 10-stage photomultiplier tube will have a gain of approximately:
   a. 10^4
   b. 4^9
   c. 4^{10}
   d. 40
   e. 400

4. Which of the following is used in TLD?
   a. Barium fluorochloride
   b. Cadmium tungstate
   c. Calcium tungstate
   d. Lithium fluoride
   e. Polyester

5. Which of the following detectors can be used to identify an unknown gamma emitter?
   a. Geiger-Müller counter
   b. Ionization chamber
   c. Lithium fluoride
   d. Scintillation detector
   e. Photographic emulsion

6. Which of the following normally operates in the rate mode?
   a. A proportional counter
   b. A thermoluminescence dosimeter
   c. An ion chamber
   d. Photographic emulsion
   e. Photoluminescence dosimeter

7. Operation in which region of a gas-filled chamber results in the lowest output?
   a. Continuous discharge
   b. Geiger-Müller region
   c. Ionization chamber
   d. Proportional
   e. Recombination

8. The resolving time of a radiation detector is the time required:
   a. For the meter to respond
   b. To detect sequential ionizations
   c. To identify different types of radiation
   d. To read the meter
   e. To reset the meter

9. The amount of light emitted by a scintillation phosphor is proportional to what feature of photon energy?
   a. Absorbed
   b. Attenuated
   c. Incident
   d. Scattered
   e. Transmitted

10. In thermoluminescence dosimetry, a plot of output intensity versus temperature is called a:
    a. Glow curve
    b. Glow worm
    c. Pulse height
    d. Pulse height analysis
    e. Pulse height spectrum

11. Which of the following statements correctly applies to the voltage response plot of the ideal gas-filled detector?
    a. Instrument sensitivity is highest in the Geiger-Müller region.
    b. The ionization region is the most sensitive.
    c. The lowest voltage of operation corresponds to the Geiger-Müller region.
    d. Voltage is higher in the proportional region than in the Geiger-Müller region.
    e. The curve has three distinct regions.

12. Which of the following is a gas-filled detector?
    a. Film badge
    b. Geiger-Müller counter
    c. Recombination chamber
    d. Scintillation counter
    e. Thermoluminescent dosimeter

13. When an accurate measurement of radiation exposure is made in the air, which should be used?
    a. Film badge
    b. Geiger-Müller counter
    c. Ionization chamber
    d. Scintillation detector
    e. TLD

14. Which of the following is characteristic of a Geiger-Müller counter?
    a. For laboratory use only
    b. Measures counts per minute
    c. Measures integrated radioactivity
    d. Useful personal monitor
    e. Wide range (0.01–100 mGy/h)

15. Which of the following is characteristic of scintillation detectors that are used as survey instruments?
    a. Can detect individual photons
    b. Are independent of energy
    c. Need extremely high voltage
    d. Suffer from saturation effects
    e. Have very low detection efficiency

16. Compared with Geiger-Müller counters, scintillation counters:
    a. Are more sensitive to gamma rays
    b. Are sensitive to beta particles
    c. Have a lower background counting rate
    d. Make better occupational radiation monitors
    e. Will count longer

17. The signal detector of a gas-filled radiation detector is the:
    a. Central electrode
    b. Chamber case
    c. Ionization region
    d. Planchet
    e. Scintillation crystal

Worksheet 39-1
Patient Radiation Dose
Reduction of Unnecessary Patient Dose

In diagnostic radiology, radiation control procedures are designed to maintain patient radiation dose ALARA (as low as reasonably achievable) while producing quality images. This requires measurement and estimation of patient dose.

Patient dose is expressed in four ways. The first, **entrance skin dose (ESD)**, can be measured easily. One can directly measure the output intensity of an x-ray unit at the source-to-skin distance, or one can position dosimeters such as those used in thermoluminescence dosimetry on the skin of the patient for direct measurement during examination.

The second method of expressing patient dose is to state the radiation dose to the bone marrow. This dose, of course, cannot be measured directly; it must be computed from phantom exposures and skin measurements. The marrow dose is used to estimate the population **mean marrow dose**, which is considered to be an indication of the leukemogenic radiation hazard.

A third method of expressing patient dose relates to potential genetic effects and usually to gonad dose. Gonad dose can be directly measured in males, but it can only be estimated in females. This is an important patient dose quantity because it is used to estimate the **genetically significant dose (GSD)**. The GSD is the dose of radiation that, if received by the entire population, would result in the same dose to the gene pool that is actually received by those irradiated.

Finally, tissue radiation dose is a method that takes into account the sensitivity of various organs in the body. This dose is heavily dependent on the tissue being exposed to radiation and the type of procedure being done.

EXERCISES

1. The GSD from medical radiation exposure depends on all of the following *except* the:
   a. Average gonad dose per examination
   b. Future childbearing expectancy of the population during any given year
   c. Number of people examined during any given year
   d. Occupational exposure
   e. Total population

2. Which of the following units is *most* appropriate when patient dose is expressed?
   a. Coulombs/kilogram
   b. Gray
   c. Rem
   d. Becquerel
   e. Sievert

3. Which of the following is *most* important in determining patient dose during radiography?
   a. Grid ratio
   b. SID
   c. Single-phase or three-phase power
   d. Size of the field exposed
   e. Size of the focal spot

4. Which of the following procedures might result in an ESE that exceeds 100 mGy_a?
   a. 5 minutes of fluoroscopy
   b. A 10-minute sonogram
   c. A mammogram
   d. An intravenous pyelogram
   e. Spiral CT

5. The GSD is:
   a. A radiation dose that will produce chromosomal aberrations
   b. An index of radiation received by the gene pool
   c. Determined from A-bomb survivor data
   d. The radiation dose is considered to be the threshold for genetic mutations
   e. Used to predict the level of genetic damage

6. The mean marrow dose is:
   a. Approximately 2 mGy/yr
   b. Considered an important indicator of somatic radiation hazard
   c. Greater than the gonad dose for examinations of the abdomen and pelvis
   d. An index of radiation response
   e. That which results in leukemia

7. In the United States, the GSD from medical radiation exposure is approximately:
   a. 0.05 mGy_t/y
   b. 0.2 mGy_t/y
   c. 0.5 mGy_t/y
   d. 2 mGy_t/y
   e. 5 mGy_t/y

8. If a 26-year-old female undergoes a KUB (radiography of the *k*idneys, *u*reters, and *b*ladder) examination, which will be the highest?
   a. Bone marrow dose
   b. Gonad dose
   c. Kidney dose
   d. Mean marrow dose
   e. Skin dose

9. Which of the following examinations results in the highest ESD?
   a. Abdomen
   b. Cervical spine
   c. Lateral chest
   d. Lateral skull
   e. Lumbar spine

10. In radiography of the lumbar spine, which of the following techniques would provide the *least* patient ESD?
    a. 84 kVp, 100 mAs
    b. 90 kVp, 100 mAs
    c. 95 kVp, 50 mAs
    d. 95 kVp, 100 mAs
    e. 84 kVp, 200 mAs

11. Medical radiation dose to the total population:
    a. Is nonsignificant
    b. Is stable in time
    c. Has greatly increased in the past few decades
    d. Has been proven to increase cancer risk
    e. Has decreased over the past few decades

12. Which has the highest tissue sensitivity to radiation?
    a. Liver
    b. Skin
    c. Thyroid
    d. Bone marrow
    e. Feet

13. Which of the following is the most likely to produce a skin burn due to ionizing radiation?
    a. Chest x-ray
    b. Interventional cardiology procedure
    c. Head CT
    d. Chest CT
    e. Head MRI

14. Digital radiographic tomosynthesis provides superior ____________ over traditional radiography.
    a. Spatial resolution
    b. Image contrast
    c. Radiation dose
    d. Brightness
    e. Income

15. The highest percentage of active bone marrow in adults can be found in which of the following places?
    a. Head
    b. Ribs
    c. C-spine
    d. Lower limb girdle
    e. Sacrum

16. Skin dose in fluoroscopy procedures is difficult to estimate primarily because of which of the following?
    a. Long exposure times
    b. High kVp
    c. Changes in angle and collimation
    d. Patient thickness
    e. Changes in anatomy

Worksheet 40-1
CT Patient Radiation Dose

In the past three decades, the use of computed tomography (CT) in medical imaging has greatly improved the quality of life and increased the life spans of many people. Due to the significant advantages CT provides in the diagnosis of diseases, the quantity of CT scanners and CT scans has also increased greatly in number. This is why it is important to be aware of CT dose and methods to keep it as low as reasonably achievable while maintaining appropriate image quality.

CT variables such as pitch, kVp, mAs, and slice thickness should all be optimized based on the patient size and indication. Additionally, dose reduction techniques such as dose modulation and iterative reconstruction should be implemented when possible to further aid in dose reduction related to CT scanning.

EXERCISES

1. Which of the following statements is *true* about CT dose?
   a. Effective dose depends on the age of the patient and the anatomy that is exposed to radiation.
   b. The peak skin dose is of primary importance, and factors such as beam angle affect its calculation.
   c. Entrance skin exposure in CT is measured regularly.
   d. CT scanners with more slices have a higher dose.
   e. CT dose is similar to the dose from an x-ray examination.

2. CT accounts for what percentage of patients effective dose?
   a. 10%
   b. 30%
   c. 50%
   d. 70%
   e. 0%

3. CT tissue dose is approximately equal to:
   a. The average x-ray tissue dose
   b. The average fluoroscopic tissue dose
   c. The average MRI tissue dose
   d. Three years of background radiation tissue dose
   e. Five years of background radiation tissue dose

4. Which of the following would be most likely to produce the highest radiation dose in a head CT scan?
   a. 64-slice helical CT
   b. 16-slice CT
   c. Step-and-shoot CT
   d. 128-slice helical CT
   e. Fluoroscopy

5. If all other factors remain the same and there is no dose modulation, a/an ________ in kVp in CT will ________ the patient dose.
   a. Increase; decrease
   b. Decrease; increase
   c. Increase; increase
   d. Increase; not change
   e. Decrease; not change

6. CT systems today are primarily all:
   a. First-generation CT scanners
   b. Second-generation CT scanners
   c. Third-generation CT scanners
   d. Fourth-generation CT scanners
   e. Fifth-generation CT scanners

7. $CTDI_{vol}$ is a measure of?
   a. CT dose to a patient
   b. CT dose to a 16 or 32 cm test object
   c. Skin dose to a patient
   d. CT lung dose
   e. CT orbital dose

8. The dose length product (DLP) is a product of which of the following?
   a. $CTDI_{center}$ and $CTDI_{periphery}$
   b. $CTDI_{vol}$ and slice thickness
   c. Slice thickness and patient thickness
   d. Patient size and $CTDI_{vol}$
   e. $CTDI_{vol}$ and the scan length in cm

9. Which of the following gives a CT dose that is corrected for patient size?
   a. Absorbed dose
   b. $CTDI_{vol}$
   c. DLP
   d. SSDE
   e. Exposure

10. Why does a thicker beam width in CT typically lead to a reduction in radiation dose?
    a. Less total penumbra effect
    b. Lower kVp is possible
    c. The mAs is typically lower
    d. Fewer photons are needed
    e. Shorter scan time

11. Which of the following is a typical $CTDI_{vol}$ value for a head CT?
    a. 20 mGy
    b. 40 mSv
    c. 60 mGy
    d. 30 mSv
    e. 30 mGy

12. Effective dose gives which of the following information?
    a. Absorbed dose from CT
    b. Equivalent whole body dose
    c. $CTDI_{vol}$
    d. Exposure to the thyroid
    e. DLP

13. A typical effective dose in a CT examination could be which of the following?
    a. 100 mSv
    b. 100 mGy
    c. 10 mGy
    d. 20 mGy
    e. 10 mSv

14. Overranging causes?
    a. Higher kVp values
    b. Poor dose modulation
    c. Improved dose modulation
    d. Reduced radiation dose
    e. Increased radiation dose

15. If imaging parameters are consistent, but a change is made to reduce noise, which of the following occurs?
    a. Lower cancer risk
    b. Increased patient dose
    c. Reduce cost
    d. Increased beam width
    e. Decreased image quality

16. Dose modulation should almost always be used when scanning patients in CT because which of the following is true?
    a. It will greatly improve image quality.
    b. It will increase patient dose by at least 30%.
    c. It will decrease patient dose by up to 50%.
    d. The patient will feel more rested after the exam.
    e. Diagnosis will be more accurate

17. Which of the following is used to take measurements that allow for the calculation of $CTDI_{vol}$?
    a. Geiger-Mueller counter
    b. Sodium iodide probe
    c. Pencil ionization chamber
    d. Solid state dosimeter
    e. Multimeter

18. The radiation beam in CT is described as a:
    a. Cone beam
    b. Square beam
    c. Parallelogram
    d. Circle beam
    e. Area beam

19. The central axis dose in CT is approximately what percentage of the entrance skin dose?
    a. 100%
    b. 200%
    c. 10%
    d. 20%
    e. 50%

Worksheet 41-1
Patient Radiation Dose Management

Exposure to radiation during diagnostic radiology, whether as a patient or as a technologist, is extremely low. Nevertheless, because of the increased sensitivity of the fetus to radiation, the portion of a radiation safety program that deals with x-rays and pregnancy requires some extra effort.

Pregnant patients should be alerted by information posted in the waiting area. Pregnant technologists should be assigned a second personnel radiation monitor with instructions that it be worn under the protective apron at waist level.

If, after a radiologic examination, a patient is found to be pregnant, the extent of the examination should be reviewed, the fetal dose should be estimated, and the time of gestation at which the dose was delivered should be determined. **Termination of pregnancy is rarely indicated**. However, should the fetal dose exceed 250 mGyt, the risk of latent injury may justify a therapeutic termination of pregnancy.

The pregnant technologist should inform her supervisor as soon as she knows of her condition so that a second monitor can be provided. The dose limit for the fetus is 0.5 mSv/month.

EXERCISES

1. If an anteroposterior (AP) examination of the abdomen results in an entrance skin exposure (ESE) of 2.20 mGya, the approximate fetal dose will be:
   a. 0.05 mGy_t
   b. 0.5 mGy_t
   c. 0.770 mGy_t
   d. 0.2 mGy_t
   e. 0.03 mGy_t

2. When a second radiation monitor is provided to a pregnant radiologic technologist:
   a. It should be worn at the collar position.
   b. It should be worn outside the apron at waist level.
   c. It should be worn under the apron at waist level.
   d. She should alternate wearing the two.
   e. She should wear both under the apron at waist level.

3. What could a radiologic technologist do to reduce the radiation dose to the fetus of a pregnant patient?
   a. Decrease kVp and increase mAs
   b. Increase object-to-image receptor distance (OID)
   c. Increase source-to-image receptor distance (SID) and mAs
   d. Reduce exposure time
   e. Use specific area shields if appropriate

4. A patient is to undergo a radiographic examination because of low back pain. As she is being positioned, she asks whether this will affect her current pregnancy. What should the radiologic technologist do?
   a. Ignore the patient.
   b. Reassure her and proceed with the examination.
   c. Refuse to do the examination.
   d. Seek advice from the radiologist before proceeding.
   e. Use a high-kVp technique and a gonad shield.

5. Which of the following techniques results in the lowest exposure to the fetus?
   a. 60 kVp, 80 ms, 100 mA
   b. 85 kVp, 200 ms, 300 mA
   c. 90 kVp, 200 ms, 100 mA
   d. 100 kVp, 200 ms, 100 mA
   e. 120 kVp, 100 ms, 100 mA (higher kVP and lower mAs)

6. After a skull series, a brain scan, a barium enema, and an intravenous pyelogram, it is discovered that the patient is pregnant. What is the correct course of action?
   a. Estimate the fetal dose.
   b. Do nothing.
   c. Perform a hysterosalpingogram.
   d. Reassure the patient and send her home.
   e. Terminate the pregnancy.

7. Radiation dose to the fetus from radiographic procedures is usually:
   a. <0.01 Gy_t
   b. 0.02 to 0.04 Gy_t
   c. 0.05 to 0.1 Gy_t
   d. 0.1 to 0.2 Gy_t
   e. >0.2 Gy_t

8. What effects of diagnostic radiation exposure are possible in a newborn (from imaging after birth or from intrauterine radiation)?
   a. Chromosomal aberrations
   b. Extrauterine growth retardation
   c. Intrauterine growth restriction
   d. Microcephaly
   e. Neonatal death

9. A patient who is 2 months pregnant is to undergo intravenous pyelography. Which of the following is correct?
   a. No more than two radiographs should be made.
   b. Normal precautions are adequate because fetal damage is least likely during this period of gestation.
   c. A pregnancy test should be ordered first.
   d. The examination should be delayed if possible.
   e. The possibility of spontaneous abortion is high.

10. The greatest nonlethal radiation hazard to an embryo or fetus occurs:
    a. During the first 2 weeks of gestation
    b. At 2 to 10 weeks of gestation
    c. At 8 to 15 weeks of gestation
    d. During the second trimester
    e. During the third trimester

11. The National Council on Radiation Protection and Measurements recommends a therapeutic abortion if the fetal dose exceeds:
    a. 0.01 Gy_t
    b. 0.05 Gy_t
    c. 0.1 Gy_t
    d. 0.25 Gy_t
    e. No recommendation is made.

12. In pelvic radiography, a dose to the shielded female gonads is primarily due to the:
    a. Characteristic x-rays released by high-atomic-number atoms in the pelvis
    b. Internally scattered x-rays
    c. Leakage radiation and air scatter
    d. Secondary electrons scattered out of the x-ray field
    e. X-rays scattered from nearby objects

13. When a radiologic technologist becomes pregnant, she should be:
    a. Counseled on proper radiation safety
    b. Fired
    c. Given a temporary leave of absence
    d. Given an additional lead apron
    e. Reassigned to nonfluoroscopy work

14. For a pregnant radiologic technologist, required radiation protection practice includes which of the following?
    a. Assignment to a low-exposure job
    b. No fluoroscopy
    c. Providing an additional apron
    d. Providing two radiation monitors
    e. Use of a gonad shield

15. Which of the following is needed to calculate the dose received by a fetus after a radiographic procedure?
    a. Fetal sex
    b. Gestation period
    c. Grid ratio
    d. Image receptor speed
    e. X-ray output

16. The fetal dose below which termination of pregnancy need not be considered is approximately:
    a. 0.02 Gy_t
    b. 0.05 Gy_t
    c. 0.1 Gy_t
    d. 0.2 Gy_t
    e. 0.5 Gy_t

17. To protect a patient from low-energy photons, one should use which of the following?
    a. Cone
    b. Increased SID
    c. Small focal spot
    d. Increased filtration
    e. Tighter collimation

18. Which of the following tools helps to reduce patient dose during radiographic examination?
    a. Post-process collimation
    b. Calipers
    c. Filtration
    d. Grids
    e. Tomography

19. In the production of an acceptable radiograph, patient dose increases as ___________ increases.
    a. Added filtration
    b. The grid ratio
    c. Collimation
    d. Focal spot
    e. The SID

20. If the skin dose from a single CT image is compared with that from multiple images:
    a. The dose will be the same for both.
    b. The multiple-image dose will be proportionally higher in relation to the number of images.
    c. The multiple-image dose will be slightly higher.
    d. The multiple-image dose will be twice as high.
    e. The single-image dose will be slightly higher.

21. Which of the following devices is designed specifically for patient protection purposes?
    a. Dental pointer cone with an integral diaphragm
    b. Fixed diaphragm
    c. Positive beam-limiting system
    d. Fluoroscopic shutters
    e. 2.5 mm Al added filtration

Worksheet 42-1 Occupational Radiation Dose Management

The dose limit (DL) applies only to occupationally exposed persons—not to patients. The DL is the dose of radiation below which the probability of harmful somatic or genetic effects is negligibly small, even when the DL is received each year of a working career.

Personnel monitoring is a program designed to measure the occupational exposure of workers. The quantity measured is the dose equivalent (DE) and the unit of DE is the sievert (rem).

Fluoroscopy is responsible for nearly all occupational radiation exposure among radiology personnel. Consequently, fluoroscopy requires maximum care with attention to good radiation safety practices. When a protective apron is worn, the monitor should be positioned above the apron and the collar region.

EXERCISES

1. The approximate average annual occupational exposure received by a radiologic technologist rarely exceeds:
   a. 5 mSv/year
   b. 50 mSv/year
   c. 25 mSv/year
   d. 10 mSv/year
   e. 30 mSv/year

2. Which of the following should *not* be part of a personnel radiation monitoring program?
   a. Film badges
   b. Optically stimulated luminescence
   c. Photoluminescence dosimetry
   d. Routine blood examination
   e. Thermoluminescence dosimeter (TLD)

3. To reduce occupational exposure during mobile x-ray examination:
   a. The patient should be given a film badge.
   b. The patient should be given a protective apron.
   c. The radiographic tube head should have a photoluminescence dosimeter.
   d. The radiologic technologist should wear a personnel monitor.
   e. The radiologic technologist should wear a protective apron.

4. In the evaluation of a personnel monitoring report:
   a. Beta radiation is considered to contribute to the whole-body dose.
   b. Extremity dose is the most limiting.
   c. Lens dose is most limiting.
   d. The skin dose is considered the sum of the whole-body dose and the extremity dose.
   e. Whole-body dose is usually the highest.

5. Which of the following is required on the personnel monitoring report?
   a. Activity in millicuries
   b. Birth date
   c. Cumulative annual skin exposure
   d. Occupational position
   e. Position of monitor

6. Recommendations proposed for mobile x-ray imaging systems state that the exposure cord length should be at least:
   a. 1 m
   b. 1.5 m
   c. 2 m
   d. 3 m
   e. 5 m

7. Personnel monitoring is required:
   a. For all radiology employees
   b. Only for radiologic technologists and radiologists
   c. When a pregnant patient is deliberately examined
   d. When it is likely that one will receive $^{1}/_{10}$ the DL
   e. When it is likely that one will receive the DL

8. A nurse is 3 ft to the patient's side during a portable chest x-ray exposure. What is likely to be her exposure?
   a. <0.01 mGy_a
   b. 0.01 to 0.05 mGy_a
   c. 0.05 to 0.1 mGy_a
   d. 0.1 to 0.25 mGy_a
   e. >0.25 mGy_a

9. Which of the following personnel monitors can be worn the longest?
   a. Film badge
   b. Geiger-Müller tube
   c. Pocket ionization chamber
   d. Scintillation monitor
   e. TLD device

10. During fluoroscopy, the personnel radiation monitor should be worn:
   a. Anywhere; it really does not matter
   b. At waist level, outside the apron
   c. At waist level, under the apron
   d. On the chest
   e. On the collar, outside the apron

11. Personnel monitoring must be conducted at least:
   a. Every 2 weeks
   b. Monthly
   c. Every 2 months
   d. Quarterly
   e. Annually

12. A 0.5 mm Pb equivalent apron attenuates a 75 kVp x-ray beam by approximately:
   a. 10%
   b. 30%
   c. 70%
   d. 90%
   e. 99%

13. Which of the following people is the *most* appropriate choice to hold a patient during a radiologic examination?
   a. Nurse
   b. Orderly
   c. Radiologic technologist
   d. Radiology secretary
   e. Relative

14. Which of the following statements about the use of protective apparel is *true?*
   a. Aprons are required even when a technologist is behind a protective barrier.
   b. During pregnancy, two aprons should be worn.
   c. Gloves should be worn by all who hold patients during the x-ray examination.
   d. It is unnecessary during mobile radiography.
   e. It is unnecessary while in the room during computed tomography.

15. Which of the following personnel radiation monitors is most sensitive?
   a. Film badge
   b. Geiger-Müller tube
   c. Pocket ionization chamber
   d. Scintillation detector
   e. TLD device

16. Which of the following is an advantage of film over TLD for personnel monitoring?
   a. Can be reused
   b. Can be used for longer periods
   c. Is cheaper
   d. Is less energy-dependent in the diagnostic range
   e. Is less sensitive to heat and humidity

17. Personnel monitoring of the extremities is necessary:
   a. During angio/interventional procedures
   b. During contrast injections
   c. During mobile radiography
   d. When the dose to the hands may exceed $^{1}/_{10}$ the DL
   e. When the dose to the hands may exceed 50 mSv/year (5000 mrem/year)

18. Filters are used in film badges to:
   a. Correct for film fog
   b. Correct for length of wear
   c. Estimate radiation energy
   d. Identify the wearer
   e. Increase the sensitivity

19. For radiologists, protective eyewear:
   a. Is unnecessary
   b. Must be used for C-arm fluoroscopy
   c. Must be used with fluoroscopy with no protective curtain
   d. Must have 0.5 mm Pb equivalent shielding
   e. Must have side shields for scatter